RESTAURANT LOVERS' LOVERS' FAT GRAM COUNTER

THE
RESTAURANT LOVERS' FAT GRAM COUNTER

Kalia Doner

BERKLEY BOOKS, NEW YORK

THE RESTAURANT LOVERS'
FAT GRAM COUNTER

A Berkley Book / published by arrangement with
the author and with Hill Nutrition Associates.

PRINTING HISTORY
Berkley edition / August 1995

ISBN: 0-425-14919-6

BERKLEY®
Berkley Books are published by The Berkley Publishing Group,
200 Madison Avenue, New York, New York 10016.
BERKLEY and the "B" design
are trademarks belonging to Berkley Publishing Corporation.

PRINTED IN THE UNITED STATES OF AMERICA

10   9   8   7   6   5   4   3   2   1

ACKNOWLEDGMENTS

Thanks to Lynn and Bill Hill of Hill Nutrition in Stuart, Florida, for their patient and precise analysis of the nutritional content of the recipes. They were able to sleuth out the most obscure data—from ackee to zabaglione. I'm also grateful to Frank M. of Citerella Fish and Andrew Rossi of Citerella Meat in New York City for their assistance.

To my editor, Heather Jackson, and my agent, Regula Noetzli at the Charlotte Sheedy Agency, my thanks for their good humor, insight, and support.

CONTENTS

INTRODUCTION

The average American eats in restaurants more than 200 times a year. That's 200 meals where there's no way to know the nutritional content of the food. *The Restaurant Lovers' Fat Gram Counter* is the first book to provide that information.

Based on recipes from some of the best restaurants in the country, the counter reveals the nutritional content of the foods you love: Italian, Chinese, Mexican, French, German, Greek, Thai, Vietnamese, Indian, Caribbean, South American, Spanish, African and Middle Eastern.

The counter offers you:

• Easy-to-read menu charts that present the calorie, fat, protein, sodium, carbohydrate, and cholesterol content of many appetizers, entrees, side dishes, condiments, sauces, and desserts.

• A serving-guide to help you determine how many servings you get in an average restaurant order.

• Advice on how to put together a healthful meal; how to talk to your waiter; and how to get special requests, with no fuss.

• Suggestions for high- medium- and low-calorie dinner orders from each cuisine.

A Basic Foods section lists the nutritional information for common meats, fish, vegetables, fruits, dairy and sweets. Use the basic food information combined with sauce and seasoning items listed in particular cuisines. This allows you to figure out calorie, fat and cholesterol contents of menu items not listed in the charts.

The counter will show you how to enjoy your favorite foods, such as spaghetti marinara, chicken fajitas, sushi, even a frosty Bahama Mama without worry. And it will alert you to potential "problem" foods: You'll discover that those cold sesame noodles you gobble down as an appetizer, *before* you eat a Chinese dinner, have over 1,000 calories and 66 grams of fat—more fat than many people should eat in a day. And that even broiled fish can tip the scale. We analyzed a famous chef's recipe for a 4-ounce filet of red snapper garnished with scallop mousse and it weighed in with 1,200 calories.

The Restaurant Lovers' Fat Gram Counter. . . don't eat out without it!

Test Your Menu Know-how

1. What contains the most fat?
  a) One dinner-sized Greek salad
  b) Beef Wellington—6 oz. meat in a puff pastry shell
  c) Italian cheesecake—1/6 of a 9" pie

2. You need to eat:
  a) At least six servings rice, pasta or bread a day
  b) Two to three servings fruit a day
  c) Three to five servings vegetables a day

3. Total cholesterol consumption for a day should be no more than:
  a) 200 mg
  b) 250 mg
  c) 300 mg

4. What has more sodium?
  a) Sweet and sour shrimp
  b) One beef burrito
  c) One piece spinach pie

5. The average woman who is moderately active should consume:
  a) Exactly 900 calories a day
  b) No more than 1,600 calories a day
  c) At least 2,000 calories a day

6. Which method of cooking is most healthful?
   a) Grilling
   b) Steaming
   c) Broiling

7. What's the best way to ask for a dish that is not on the menu?
   a) Call ahead and alert the chef
   b) Insist the waiter bring the chef to your table to discuss preparation
   c) Ask the waiter when it's your turn to order

Answers:

1. B. One serving of beef Wellington has 124 grams of fat, two to three times a day's allotment. A Greek salad has 50 grams and Italian cheesecake, 30 grams.

2. A, B, and C. You don't improve your health by eating too little. The key to health is eating moderate quantities of a wide variety of food every day.

3. It depends on whom you ask. The government's cholesterol recommendation is 300 mg. However, some nutritionists recommend you cut it to 200 to 250 mg a day.

4. B. A beef burrito has 879 mg sodium. Sweet and sour shrimp, 616 mg; spinach pie, 417 mg. Daily intake should be less than 2,400 mg.

5. C. 2,000 calories to maintain weight. If you exercise at least four hours a week (walk, jog, bicycle, lift weights, swim, play tennis) you can eat more than you may think.

6. All three can be healthful—if the chef doesn't add excess oil or butter. For grilled or broiled foods, ask that they be basted with lemon or lime juice, basic tomato sauce, or mustard in place of oil. For steamed foods, ask that oil or butter not be added.

7. All of the above—depending on the situation. You may call ahead if you're uncomfortable discussing your special requests in front of your dinner companions. These days most restaurants are relaxed about special requests. If you ask your waiter for dishes prepared without sauces or broiled instead of fried, it's usually no problem. As for getting the cook out to your table—there are places where it's so fancy or so casual that you can pull it off, but most of the time, leave the chef alone. He's got work to do. Your waiter can transmit your message.

Fat Facts:

The USDA recommends we limit fat intake to 30 percent of our daily calories.

Sedentary people, who should eat about 1,600 to 2,000 calories a day, should take in between 480 and 600 calories (53 to 66 grams) from fat. Moderately active women, eating 2,000 to 2,200 calories a day, should take in no more than 660 calories (73 grams) from fat. Moderately active men, eating 2,700 to 3,000 calories a day, should limit fat intake to 900 calories (100 grams). (Many nutritionists think these figures are too high and set a target of 25 percent.)

Fat is not all bad, however. Some types of oils—polyunsaturated and monounsaturated—help the body clear heart-stopping cholesterol from the bloodstream. When possible, order food prepared with the most healthful varieties of oil, but be moderate in their use at all times.

Okay oils: These are highest in unsaturated fats: canola, almond, safflower, corn, olive, walnut, and sesame. Olive oil is highest in monounsaturated fats, which are the most effective in removing harmful cholesterol from the bloodstream.

Not-so-okay oils: These are loaded with saturated fat—the fat that prevents the body from clearing cholesterol from the bloodstream: coconut, palm kernel, butter, cocoa butter, and cottonseed. Coconut oil is 92 percent saturated fat. Canola oil is only 7 percent.

FLASH! One gram of fat = 9 calories.

Watch Out for Hidden Fat!

Salad dressings. One tablespoon of Roquefort dressing has 8 grams of fat ... and most people use at least three times that on a small salad. One tablespoon of vinaigrette has even more—10 grams. But low-calorie Italian has less than 2 grams and a tablespoon of balsamic vinegar has none.

Chips. Tortilla chips, potato chips and those funny little crisps at Chinese restaurants are loaded with fat—in fact that's almost all they are. Half of the calories in corn chips are from fat.

Sauces. There's nothing wrong with sauces. They make the meal. But their nutritional content varies enormously: 1/4 cup marinara sauce may have 70 calories and 7 grams fat; 1/4 cup Alfredo sauce may have 204 calories and 21 grams fat. The lowest-fat sauces are: marinara, primavera, puttanesca, arrabbiata, white clam sauce, and all Mexican salsas.

Ten Ways to Estimate the Fat Content of Any Dish You Order

If you are curious about the fat content of a dish that's not on our menu analysis, you can make an educated guess.

✖ Every ounce of lean red meat (not hamburger) you eat has approximately 9 grams fat and 22–25 mg cholesterol.

✖ Every ounce of skinless chicken has around 2 grams fat and 24–25 mg cholesterol.

✖ Every ounce of filet of sole has around 0.37 grams fat and 14 mg cholesterol.

✖ Every tablespoon of vegetable oil adds about 14 grams fat but no cholesterol.

✖ Every tablespoon of butter adds about 12 grams fat and 33 mg cholesterol.

✖ Assume that frying adds approximately 200 calories to any entree serving. If the food is breaded, add at least another 100 calories.

✖ An egg in any sauce or dish will add an extra 6 grams fat and 213 mg cholesterol.

✖ A tablespoon of sour cream in a sauce or used as a topping adds 3 grams fat and 13 mg cholesterol to your meal.

✖ Assume that anything that looks "healthy" but tastes "sinful" is. Add at least 10 grams fat and 20 mg cholesterol per bite.

✕ Every glass of wine adds approximately 85 calories, but no fat or cholesterol to your meal.

Cholesterol Counting

The USDA recommends limiting cholesterol intake to 300 mg a day. That's the equivalent of 1 1/2 eggs; one slice of quiche Lorraine, a cheese calzone, about half an entree-sized squid salad, or three Chinese crepes filled with mu shu pork.

How to Order Healthful Food. . . Even if It's Not on the Menu

Most cuisines employ a range of cooking styles—even French restaurants offer heart-stopping sauces *and* healthful grilled fish, super-rich casseroles *and* exceptionally flavorful salads and vegetables. And there are very few establishments that won't go out of their way to accommodate you—if you are clear about your desires.

• Explain what you want: low calorie, low sodium, low cholesterol, or low fat.

• Ask the waiter for recommendations from the menu and explanations of how the food is prepared.

• If you want to have some item prepared differently from what is listed on the menu, explain what you want carefully and precisely.

• If none of the menu items can be adjusted as you want, talk to the waiter about having something prepared "off" the menu. You should suggest what you're looking for. Broiled or grilled fish or meat. Salad without cheese. Steamed vegetables. Food with little or no soy sauce. Try to ask all questions and make all your requests at once so the waiter doesn't have to run back and forth to ask the chef a series of questions.

• Be patient. Special dishes may take more time to prepare.

• Stick up for yourself. If you ask for steamed veggies without oil, and they arrive at the table glistening with butter, send them back.

6

If you don't want to involve your waiter in your quest for a healthful meal, skip any dish with rich sauces, fried foods, cheese, sour cream, or gravy. Instead, choose roasted and broiled game and poultry and pass on desserts. Or simply make a vow to eat only half of any serving, sharing your meal with your dinner companions or taking it home. If, for example, the restaurant serves an 8-ounce order of sauerbraten, eating only half of it eliminates around 400 calories and 30 grams of fat!

Ask Your Waiter

Whatever your approach, there are some basic questions that you can ask your waitperson to help you make wise choices.

- What kind of oil is used to fry foods?
- Is this dish fried?
- Can you make the dish without deep frying?
- Can you steam the (vegetables) or (fish)?
- Can you put the sauce on the side?
- Can I have a half order?
- Can you make the dish without cheese or cheese sauce?
- What is the sauce made with?
- Can you prepare this without the sauce?
- How large is the serving? How many ounces of beef, chicken, fish, etc. is used?
- Can you make this dish without soy sauce or MSG?

Words for the Wise

Menus provide clear clues to the way food is cooked. Feel free to indulge in those that are described as steamed, broiled, roasted, poached.

High-Salt Alert

If you must watch sodium intake, steer clear of foods that are pickled, smoked, in cocktail sauce, in broth, with soy sauce, or with MSG.

High-fat cooking techniques

Menu clues to fatty foods: parmigiana, au gratin, marinated, crispy, fried, breaded, with gravy, whipped, creamed, hollandaise, Alfredo.

Good Bite, Bad Bite

Menu Choices	Abstemious	Indulgent
Appetizers	vegetable juice, fresh fruit, shrimp or crab cocktail, grilled vegetables, oysters	creamed soup, deep-fried vegetables, cheese, wings
Salad	any greens or veggies with low-fat dressing	salad with cheese, meat, avocado, creamy dressing, eggs
Carbos	steamed rice, pasta, oven-roasted or boiled potatoes	fried or creamed rice or potatoes, stuffed pasta, cheese- or cream-based sauces
Veggies	steamed, fresh, grilled, or broiled	creamed, fried, breaded, with cheese
Main Courses	roasted (without skin), broiled, steamed, grilled, boiled, poached	fried, breaded, stuffed, with cream sauce or cheese
Desserts	fruit, sorbets and ices	everything else

How Much Is. . .

To help you judge how much you want to eat of what you've ordered, the following chart provides equivalents.

Shrimp

Medium = 31–35 shrimp per pound
Large = 21 –25 per pound
Jumbo = 6–8 per pound
Sweet water prawns = 6 per pound

Scallops

Sea scallops = 20 scallops per pound
Bay scallops = 40 per pound

Swordfish

Average steak, 1 1/4" thick = 1 pound

Mussels

20–25 per pound
1 generous quart = 2 pounds

Meat and Poultry

Quail = 7 ounces total weight
Partridge = 10 ounces total weight
One chicken breast, boneless, skinless = 8–12
    ounces
T-bone = 16–20 ounces (typical restaurant size)
Filet mignon = 8 ounces
Beef stew = 14–18 chunks per pound
Spare ribs (pork) = 12 to a rack = 2 1/2 pounds
Beef, 3 ounces = the size of a deck of cards

Tortellini

24 small cheese tortellini = 3 ounces
12 large = 3 ounces

Capellini (Angel Hair)

4 ounces = approximately 2 cups cooked

Linguini

4 ounces = approximately 2 cups cooked

Vegetables and Fruit

Broccoli, 21 florets = 1 pound
Tomato, 2 1/2" diameter = 10 ounces
Asparagus, 32 thin stalks = 1 pound
Strawberries, 24 average size = 1 pound
Black olives, large, 70 = 1 pound

CHINESE MENUS

CHINESE MENU SAVVY

When is a serving not a serving? When you order at a Chinese restaurant. Most menu items come with at least two, and often three or four, servings per order. That means even relatively low-calorie, low-fat dishes such as chicken chow mein become a nutritional disaster if you eat everything that's on your plate. Instead, eat one serving (amounts are indicated on the charts), and then share the rest with your dinner companions or take it home for later.

Another way to cut calories and fat is to focus the meal around rice, noodles, and vegetables. Use meat protein as an accent—eating no more than 2 or 3 ounces at a meal. (Three ounces of beef is about the size of a deck of cards.)

To limit sodium intake, order items without MSG and little or no soy sauce. Avoid soups. Rely on sweet and spicy sauces for flavor.

Low(er)-fat cooking is indicated by menu descriptions such as stir fried, simmered, steamed, roasted, with bean curd (not fried), with assorted vegetables, with lobster sauce, with spicy tomato sauce, in light sauce, in oyster sauce.

Fatty cooking is indicated by menu descriptions such as fried, crispy, breaded, with egg, with peanuts or cashews, with hoisin sauce, sweet and sour (not because of the sauce, but because the meat or fish is invariably deep-fried).

Sample CHINESE DINNERS for Every Appetite

	CALORIES	FAT
❖ High-calorie meals:		
Shrimp toast (1)	66	4
Egg drop soup (1 1/2 c.)	77	4
Beef with Broccoli (1/2 c.)	272	24
Buddha's Delight		
mixed vegetables (1/3 order)	146	9
White rice (1/2 c.)	176	<1

TOTAL CALORIES: 737
Fat grams: 41

Fried wontons with shrimp filling (2)	230	20
Brown rice (1 1/3 c.)	288	2
Eggplant, Szechuan style (3 oz.)	187	18
Crispy almond chicken (1/4 lb.)	377	25

TOTAL CALORIES: 1,082
Fat grams: 65

Deep-fried whole fish with spicy		
tomato sauce (2 1/2 lbs.)	2,135	101
White Rice (1 1/3 c.)	353	<1
Steamed spinach (1/2 c.)	21	<1

TOTAL CALORIES: 2,509
Fat grams: 102

❖ Medium-calorie meals:		
Steamed pork and vegetable bun (1)	151	6
Shrimp with snow peas, stir-fried		
(3 oz., or 5-6 medium, shrimp)	355	29

TOTAL CALORIES: 506
Fat grams: 35

Egg drop soup (1 1/2 c.)	77	4
Lemon Chicken (1 c., with		
3 oz. chicken)	338	14
White rice (1/2 c.)	176	<1

TOTAL CALORIES: 591
Fat grams: 18

	CALORIES	FAT
Sweet and sour shrimp (5 large)	350	16
White rice (1/2 c.)	176	<1

TOTAL CALORIES: 526
Fat grams: 16

❖ Low-calorie meals:

Steamed fish with black bean sauce (1/4 lb.)	253	14
White rice (1/4 c.)	88	<1

TOTAL CALORIES: 341
Fat grams: 14

Dumplings with pork filling, fried (4)	252	16
White rice (1/2 c.)	176	<1

TOTAL CALORIES: 428
Fat grams: 16

Steamed pork and vegetable bun (1)	151	6
Hot and sour soup (1 1/2 c.)	233	12

TOTAL CALORIES: 384
Fat grams: 18

CHINESE MENUS

	Calories	Fat	Sodium	Protein	Carbos	Cholesterol	% Calories
		(g)	(mg)	(g)	(g)	(mg)	from Fat
APPETIZERS							
Barbecued Pork— Cantonese. 4 oz. meat, or ten 1/4" strips	284	20 g	509 mg	16 g	8 g	72 mg	63%
Cold Sesame Noodles—Szechuan. 1/4 lb. noodles—half of most restaurant orders. This recipe has 2.5 oz. chicken per serving, but that accounts for only 121 calories.	1,187	66	4,298	49	105	168	50
Dumplings							
Fried with Pork Filling—Mandarin. 1 dumpling	63	4	126	2	5	5	62
Steamed with Pork Filling— Cantonese. 1 dumpling	72	3	163	3	7	9	38
Steamed with Vegetable Filling—Szechuan. 1 dumpling	31	<1	61	<1	6	0	0
Egg Roll with Ground Pork— Mandarin. 1 roll	291	19	693	7	23	14	59
Shrimp Toast— Mandarin. 1 piece	66	4	106	3	4	17	55
Spring Rolls— Shanghai. 1 roll	306	20	682	6	25	12	51
Pork and Vegetable Buns, steamed— Mandarin. 1 bun	151	6	261	6	19	14	36

	Calories	Fat	Sodium	Protein	Carbos	Cholesterol	% Calories
		(g)	(mg)	(g)	(g)	(mg)	from Fat
Wonton with shrimp filling, Fried—Cantonese. 1 wonton	115	10 g	70 mg	2 g	5 g	18 mg	78%
SAUCES and CONDIMENTS							
Almonds, Crisp—6	72	7	<1	2	2	0	88
Chili Sauce, Hot—1 tsp.	42	5	<1	<1	<1	0	100
Duck Sauce—1 T.	50	2	255	<1	7	0	36
Garlic Sauce—1 T.	36	3	341	<1	2	0	75
Lichi—1 fresh	64	<1	n.a.	<1	16	0	4
Mustard Sauce, Hot—1 tsp.	13	1	<1	<1	<1	0	69
Soy Sauce, Regular—See Japanese section.							
Tamari—See Japanese section.							
Sweet and Sour Sauce—1 T.	34	0	114	<1	8	0	0
SOUP							
Egg Drop—1 1/2 c.	77	4	373	6	4	109	47
Hot and Sour—1 1/2 c.	233	12	695	11	21	73	46
Sizzling Rice—1 serving = 3/4 cup broth and vegetables with a rice square 3" x 1/2"	405	34	1,106	7	18	25	76
Wonton—with 5 wontons	240	8	1,162	14	27	112	34

	Calories	Fat (g)	Sodium (mg)	Protein (g)	Carbos (g)	Cholesterol (mg)	% Calories from Fat
RICE and PANCAKES							
Brown Rice— 1 1/3 c.	288	2 g	13 mg	9 g	85 g	0 mg	6%
Crispy Rice—2" square	55	<1	0	<1	10	0	13
Fried Rice, Basic— 1 c. rice. The typical restaurant portion is 2–3 cups!	433	23	**1,189**	9	47	130	48
Fried Rice— loaded with sausage, shrimp, veggies. 1 c.	541	31	**1,500**	18	46	141	52
White Rice—long grain. 1 1/3 c.	353	<1	5	2	76	0	2
Green Onion Pancake—Shanghai. 1 large piece	412	21	811	7	49	6	46
Mandarin Pancake—no eggs. One 5" piece	51	1	34	1	9	0	18
Northern-Style Pancake—made with eggs. One 10" piece	188	8	194	4	24	35	38
VEGETABLES and VEGETARIAN DISHES							
Buddha's Delight— mixed vegetables with 4 oz. tofu in light stir-fry sauce	440	27	**2,118**	19	37	0	55
Bean Curd Ma Po— Szechuan. 5 oz. tofu	447	40	**1,452**	19	6	27	81
Egg Fu Young— Cantonese. Plain, with 2 eggs	347	28	632	15	10	**425**	73

	Calories	Fat	Sodium	Protein	Carbos	Cholesterol	% Calories
		(g)	(mg)	(g)	(g)	(mg)	from Fat
Eggplant, Szechuan-Style—one serving = 1/2 large eggplant. Average restaurant order has 2 servings.	560	53 g	1834 mg	4 g	21 g	0 mg	85%
Tofu, soft—3 oz.	46	2	6	4	2	0	39
Tofu, regular—3 oz.	65	4	6	7	2	0	55
Tofu, hard—3 oz.	123	7	12	13	4	0	51
FISH							
Braised Fish with Bean Curd—Mandarin. Whitefish, carp, trout, or perch. 1 whole fish, or 1 to 1 1/2 lb.	1,266	103	4,562	59	29	144	73
Chow Mein with Shrimp—Cantonese. 1/4 lb. noodles. Restarant order may contain 1/2 lb. noodles.	668	21	1,480	29	92	179	28
Deep-Fried Whole Fish with Spicy Tomato Sauce—Shanghai. Data given for one 2 1/2 lb. red snapper; other fish are similar. If it serves four, it's not a bad choice. But for one or two, it is high in fat, sodium, and cholesterol.	2,135	101	4,586	145	149	453	43
Shrimp, butterflied, breaded, and wok-fried—*Cantonese.* 1/4 lb. shrimp	375	18	659	24	28	193	43
Shrimp with Hot Sauce—Szechuan. 8–10 medium shrimp. Most orders have 2 servings	328	24	1,479	20	9	140	66

	Calories	Fat	Sodium	Protein	Carbos	Cholesterol	% Calories
		(g)	(mg)	(g)	(g)	(mg)	from Fat
Steamed Fish with Black Bean Sauce—Cantonese. 1/4 lb. fish. Most restaurant orders are 1 whole fish, or 2 servings.	253	14 g	1,065 mg	23 g	7 g	68 mg	50%
Shrimp with Snow Peas, stir-fried—Cantonese. 5–6 med. shrimp	355	29	914	15	8	93	73
Stir-fried Shrimp with Chicken—Shanghai. 3 shrimp, 2 oz. chicken. Most restaurant orders have 2 servings.	617	41	786	41	18	136	60
Sweet and Sour Shrimp, breaded and deep-fried—Cantonese. 8 medium or 5–6 large shrimp.*	350	16	616	20	31	140	41

CHICKEN

	Calories	Fat	Sodium	Protein	Carbos	Cholesterol	% Calories
Crispy Almond Chicken—Cantonese. 1/4 lb. chicken. Most restaurant orders have about 3 servings.	377	25	1,287	29	9	79	60
Chicken Chow Mein—Mandarin. 1 1/4 c., with 1/4 lb. noodles and 2 oz. chicken. Most restaurant dishes have at least 3 generous servings.	685	22	1,446	32	89	141	29

*As with all fried foods, if not well-prepared, the shrimp retain much more oil. You may take in an additional 3 T.—that's 360 more calories and 42 more grams of fat in one serving. If it looks, feels, or tastes greasy—assume the worst.

	Calories	Fat (g)	Sodium (mg)	Protein (g)	Carbos (g)	Cholesterol (mg)	% Calories from Fat
Chicken with Black Bean Sauce— Cantonese. 6 oz. chicken thighs with bones	437	35 g	1,297 mg	25 g	5 g	113 mg	72%
Chicken with Broccoli—2 c. with 5 oz. chicken. Average restaurant order has 2 servings.	472	38	1,487	26	7	59	72
Lemon Chicken— Cantonese. 1 c., with 3 oz. chicken. Average restaurant order has 2 servings.	338	14	754	21	32	103	37
Drunk Chicken, with aspiclike sauce— Shanghai. 1/4 whole chicken, about 5 oz. meat. (If you eliminate the sauce, you eliminate most of the sodium.)	396	21	**2,279**	26	7	104	48
Mu Shu Chicken— Mandarin. Two 6" to 8" pancakes	603	34	**1,348**	26	49	193	51
PORK							
Pork Chow Mein— Cantonese. 1 1/4 c. with 2 oz. pork and 1/4 lb. noodles. Most restaurant orders have 3 servings.	746	30	1,445	29	89	148	36
Pork Lo Mein— 1 1/2 c. with 4 oz. pork. Average retaurant order has 3 servings.	432	18	1,217	25	43	77	37
Mu Shu Pork— Mandarin. Two 6" to 8" pancakes	653	40	1,339	24	49	195	55

	Calories	Fat (g)	Sodium (mg)	Protein (g)	Carbos (g)	Cholesterol (mg)	% Calories from Fat
Shredded Pork with Sweet Bean Sauce—Mandarin. 3 oz. pork. Average restaurant order has 2 servings.	371	28 g	694 mg	18 g	11 g	54 mg	68%
Spare Ribs, Peking-Style—Mandarin. 1/4 lb. ribs	399	34	542	14	10	54	77
Sweet and Sour Pork—Cantonese. 1/4 lb. pork, or 5–6 1" cubes, battered and deep-fried. (See note on deep-frying perils under Sweet and Sour Shrimp.)	490	21	894	27	47	128	39
Twice-cooked Pork—Szechuan. 1 c., with 1/4 lb. pork, green pepper, and bok choy in hot bean sauce. Average restaurant order has 2–3 servings.	531	45	595	21	9	81	76
BEEF							
Beef with Broccoli—Cantonese. 2 c. with 5 oz. beef. Average restaurant order has 2 servings.	543	47	1,493	24	7	53	78
Beef Chow Mein—Mandarin. 1 1/4 c. with 1/4 lb. noodles and 2 oz. beef. Average restaurant order has 3 to 3 1/2 c.	724	27	1,450	30	89	137	34
Curried Beef—Cantonese. 3 oz. beef	495	37	1,032	18	24	40	67

	Calories	Fat	Sodium	Protein	Carbos	Cholesterol	% Calories
		(g)	(mg)	(g)	(g)	(mg)	from Fat
Mongolian Beef— Mandarin. 3 oz. beef on fried noodles. Average restaurant order has 2 servings.	544	44 g	527 mg	22 g	14 g	53 mg	73%
Mongolian Fire Pot—Mandarin. 3 oz. beef, 3–4 shrimp, 1 oz. tofu, plus veggies and broth	591	35	**2,706**	49	20	174	53
Sesame Beef— Szechuan. 2 oz. beef. Average restaurant order has 3 servings. (Dish is sometimes battered and deep-fried, adding 200–300 calories per order.)	364	33	561	12	5	43	82
Tomato Beef with Green Peppers— Cantonese. 5 oz. or about 10–12 slices of beef.	902	73	**3,074**	34	27	79	73

ITALIAN MENUS

ITALIAN MENU SAVVY

Mediterranean cuisine is basically healthful, focusing on fresh vegetables, salads, fish, grilled and roasted meats, grains, pasta, and tomato sauces. Olive oil helps clear cholesterol out of the blood, and studies indicate that garlic is also good for the cardiovascular system. But that doesn't mean that in the hands of meat-crazy, cheese-loving Americans, Italian food can't turn into a nutritional nightmare.

• *Healthful menu items* are indicated by words such as marinara, primavera, Arrabbiata, roasted, grilled, steamed, thin crust, pasta.

• *High-fat and calorie- foods* are indicated by words such as Alfredo, carbonara, parmigiana, cheese, fried, stuffed.

Rules to Remember

• For a low-fat meal, stick with simple pasta, grilled veggies, fresh fruit, and a glass of Chianti Reserve . . . who could ask for anything more?

• Ask your waiter what type of pasta they serve: fresh? dried? egg? yolkless? no egg? Each has a different calorie, cholesterol, and fat content.

Sample ITALIAN DINNERS for Every Appetite

	CALORIES	FAT
❖ High-calorie meals		
Spaghetti marinara (appetizer-sized, or 1/2 dinner-sized)	352	14
Grilled zucchini (1 small)	118	11
Zuppa di pesce (seafood stew)	187	5
Fruit ice (1/2 c.)	130	0

TOTAL CALORIES: 787
Fat grams: 30

Calzone, sausage and cheese	1,266	81

TOTAL CALORIES: 1,266
Fat grams: 81

Arugula salad with pine nuts, and olive oil and vinegar	208	19
Steamed broccoli with butter, olive oil and parmesan cheese (1/3 c.)	280	28
Spaghetti Bolognese (1/4 lb. dried pasta with 1 c. sauce)	931	37

TOTAL CALORIES: 1,419
Fat grams: 84

❖ Medium-calorie (dinner-sized) meals

Caesar salad (dinner-sized)	150	9
Roasted chicken, with skin (1/4 chicken)	362	24

TOTAL CALORIES: 512
Fat grams: 33

Tossed salad with balsamic vinegar (dinner-sized)	33	0
Mussels steamed in white wine and butter (1 qt.)	190	11
Spaghetti marinara (side order, or 1/2 dinner-sized)	352	14

TOTAL CALORIES: 575
Fat grams: 25

	CALORIES	FAT
Eggplant parmigiana	410	29
Tossed salad with Balsamic vinegar	33	0

TOTAL CALORIES: 443
Fat grams: 29

❖ Low-calorie meals

	CALORIES	FAT
Bruschetta (1 slice)	249	17
Zuppa di pesce (seafood stew)	187	5

TOTAL CALORIES: 436
Fat grams: 22

	CALORIES	FAT
Mussels steamed in white wine and butter (1 qt.)	190	11
Broccoli with garlic and olive oil	132	9

TOTAL CALORIES: 322
Fat grams: 20

	CALORIES	FAT
Pasta primavera (2 oz. linguini, and sauce with no cream)	381	16

TOTAL CALORIES: 381
Fat grams: 16

ITALIAN MENUS

	Calories	Fat	Sodium	Protein	Carbos	Cholesterol	% Calories
		(g)	(mg)	(g)	(g)	(mg)	from Fat
APPETIZERS							
Artichoke Hearts, steamed—4 oz.	42	<1 g	80 mg	3 g	9 g	0 mg	2%
Bruschetta—1 slice (It. bread with tomato, olive oil, and seasonings)	249	17	176	4	21	0	61
Bread Sticks—1 oz.	120	2	350	4	20	0	15
Bread, Italian— 1 slice, or 1 oz.	83	<1	176	3	17	<1	2
Caponata—1/4 c.	265	24	587	2	14	0	82
Calamari, fried— 1/4 lb.	261	15	72	19	11	264	52
Clams, baked stuffed—2	162	8	381	10	11	20	44
Focaccia with rosemary and sage—1 slice	278	9	277	7	41	0	29
Mozzarella Sticks, fried—4 sm. sticks or 2 lg. ones	240	16	580	9	15	20	60
Olives, Black—1 oz. or 4–5 lg.	33	3	247	<1	2	0	82
Olives, Green— unstuffed, 1 oz. or 4–5 lg.	33	4	680	<1	<1	0	21
Zucchini, fried— 1 stick	64	2	130	2	9	16	28
SOUP							
Minestrone—1 c.	127	3	870	5	21	5	21
Stracciatella—1 c.	65	4	1,087	6	1	106	55

	Calories	Fat (g)	Sodium (mg)	Protein (g)	Carbos (g)	Cholesterol (mg)	% Calories from Fat
Pasta e Fagioli— 1 1/2 c.	443	18 g	1,186 mg	17 g	54 g	0 mg	37

PIZZA

The weight of a slice of pizza varies wildly. Some restaurants serve single slices that weigh as much as or more than 2 slices at chains such as Domino's or Pizza Hut. Data here are for slices that are 1/8 of a medium 12" pie with a moderate amount of topping

	Calories	Fat (g)	Sodium (mg)	Protein (g)	Carbos (g)	Cholesterol (mg)	% Calories from Fat
Basic Pizza Dough— 2 slices of a 12" pizza	387	9	276	10	66	0	21
Thin Crust Pizza Dough— 2 slices of a 12" pizza	230	<1	368	7	48	0	3
Cheese— 2 slices of a 12" pie, 7 oz.	492	18	940	n.a.	n.a.	34	32
Pepperoni— 2 slices of a 12" pie, 7 oz.	540	22	1127	n.a.	n.a.	42	36
Sausage— 2 slices of a 12" pie, 6 oz.	430	17	1270	n.a.	n.a.	40	36
Thin crust cheese— 2 slices of a 12" pie, 6 oz.	398	17	867	n.a.	n.a.	33	38

CALZONES

	Calories	Fat (g)	Sodium (mg)	Protein (g)	Carbos (g)	Cholesterol (mg)	% Calories from Fat
Traditional (sausage, mozzarella, ricotta)	1,266	81	1,385	54	78	287	58
Prosciutto and Cheese	900	46	2,238	51	70	236	46
Cheese (fontina, provolone, mozzarella)	1,363	87	2,129	68	77	288	57

25

	Calories	Fat (g)	Sodium (mg)	Protein (g)	Carbos (g)	Cholesterol (mg)	% Calories from Fat
ITALIAN OMELET							
Frittata with cheese—3 eggs	632	49 g	1,572 mg	42 g	4 g	820 mg	70%
HOAGIES							
Salami and provolone on 9" roll	1,350	103	3,740	42	62	49	69
Meatball hero on an 8" roll (3/4 pound of meat balls, or about 4–6 in sauce)	2,141	110	4,530	106	166	482	46
SALAD							
Arugula, Pine Nuts, and Parmesan Salad with olive oil and vinegar	208	19	103	10	3	11	82
Two-Bean Salad (cannellini and black beans)—4 oz.	319	14	1,069	13	35	0	39
Caesar Salad—1 generous portion	150	9	524	9	9	40	54
Fava bean and Pecorino Cheese—1.5 oz. serving	113	9	94	6	3	11	72
Spinach Salad with red bell peppers and cheese; oil and vinegar—side-order sized	218	23	405	3	3	5	95
Squid (Calamari) Salad—5 oz. squid	379	28	584	24	8	352	66
Tossed Salad with onions, radishes, tomato, cucumber, green pepper; no dressing	33	<1	54	2	7	0	3

	Calories	Fat	Sodium	Protein	Carbos	Cholesterol	% Calories
		(g)	(mg)	(g)	(g)	(mg)	from Fat
SALAD DRESSING							
Blue Cheese—2 T.	154	16 g	335 mg	2 g	2 g	5 mg	93%
Italian, Low-Cal—2 T.	32	3	236	<1	2	0	84
Italian, Regular—2 T.	137	14	231	<1	3	0	91
Oil and Vinegar—2 T.	140	16	<1	0	<1	0	100
Olive Oil—1 T.	119	14	0	0	0	0	100
VEGETABLES*							
Broccoli steamed and tossed with olive oil and garlic—1/4 bunch	132	9	139	7	10	4	61
Broccoli tossed with butter, olive oil, and parmesan—1/3 c.	280	28	126	5	5	20	90
Eggplant Parmigiana	410	29	619	18	24	69	64
Red Peppers, roasted—1/2 pepper	8	0	120	0	2	0	0
Grilled Zucchini with olive oil—1 sm. zucchini	118	11	28	2	6	0	84
Zucchini steamed, with pine nuts and balsamic vinegar—1/2 lb.	64	5	278	3	5	0	70

*Vegetables are a wonderful food, but added oil, cheese, and sauce escalate the calories and add cholesterol. To determine the impact of what you order look up the plain vegetables listed in the Basic Foods section and then refer to sauce, cheese, and oil information in other sections.

	Calories	Fat	Sodium	Protein	Carbos	Cholesterol	% Calories
		(g)	(mg)	(g)	(g)	(mg)	from Fat

CHEESE

	Calories	Fat	Sodium	Protein	Carbos	Cholesterol	% Calories
Bleu—1 oz.	100	8 g	395 mg	6 g	<1 g	21 mg	72%
Fontina—1 oz.	110	9	227	7	<1	33	74
Mascarpone—1 oz.	130	13	5	2	<1	35	90
Mozzarella—1 oz.	80	6	106	6	<1	22	68
Parmesan—1 T. grated	23	2	93	2	<1	4	59
Provolone—1 oz.	100	8	248	7	<1	20	72
Ricotta—1/4 c.	99	7	48	6	2	29	64
Roquefort—1 oz.	103	9	507	6	<1	25	75

SAUCES
(WITHOUT PASTA)

	Calories	Fat	Sodium	Protein	Carbos	Cholesterol	% Calories
Aioli (garlic mayonnaise)—1 T.	116	13	26	<1	<1	19	99
Alfredo—2/3 c.	563	57	513	12	2	165	91
Bolognese—1 c.	499	32	1,069	27	27	99	56
Carbonara—1 serving = 4 oz. bacon, 1/2 an egg, olive oil and about 4 oz. of grated cheeses, enough for 4 oz. pasta	372	33	675	16	1	145	80
Marinara—1 c.	283	27	324	2	10	0	86
Meat sauce—1 c.	421	32	488	16	14	55	68
Pesto (sun-dried tomatoes)—1/4 c.	250	25	520	3	6	0	90
Pesto (basil) 1/4 c.	310	30	440	6	5	10	87
Primavera, no cream—generous main course serving	171	15	257	3	7	41	79
Puttanesca—1/2 c.	130	11	473	2	8	1	76

	Calories	Fat	Sodium	Protein	Carbos	Cholesterol	% Calories
		(g)	(mg)	(g)	(g)	(mg)	from Fat
Red Clam—1 c.	333	30 g	450 mg	7 g	10 g	13 mg	81%
Three Cheese (bleu, parmesan, and romano)—1/4 c.	167	15	344	8	1	23	80
Arrabbiata—1/2 c.	114	10	234	2	7	0	79
Tomato with Cream—1 c.	370	37	437	3	11	81	89
White—1/2 c. (Used for some baked pastas and as a basis for cream and cheese sauces.)	199	15	152	5	11	48	68
White Clam—1/2 c.	120	9	310	10	1	15	68
PASTA*							

Dried Pasta
  Egg Noodles
  Fettucini, Lasagna
  Tagliatelle,
  Tagliarini—4 oz.
	432	5	24	16	81	108	10

Spinach egg noodles—4 oz.	433	5	82	17	80	108	10
Eggless Dried Macaroni (Angel Hair/Capellini, Bucatini, Conchiglie, Farfalle, Fusilli, Linguini, Penne, Rotelle, Rigatoni, Spaghetti, Spaghettini)—4 oz.	421	2	8	14	85	0	4

*Most main course servings of pasta are 4 oz., twice the size of what is called a serving on a package. Side dishes may be 2 oz. As for the data presented here—the old rule of thumb was that fresh pasta was made with egg and dried pasta could be with or without egg. Now there's fresh pasta made with no eggs or with egg whites. You never know what version you're getting unless you ask.

	Calories	Fat (g)	Sodium (mg)	Protein (g)	Carbos (g)	Cholesterol (mg)	% Calories from Fat
Fresh Egg Pasta (Angel Hair, Fettucini, Lasagne, Pappardelle, Tagliatelle—4 oz.	327	3 g	29 mg	13 g	62 g	83 mg	8%
Spinach Pasta— 4 oz.	328	2	31	13	63	83	5
Yolkless Pasta— 4 oz.	396	3	26	16	79	0	6

OTHER STARCHES

	Calories	Fat (g)	Sodium (mg)	Protein (g)	Carbos (g)	Cholesterol (mg)	% Calories from Fat
Cannelloni in cream sauce—3 med. or 2 lg. rolls	514	30	642	27	34	257	53
Gnocchi Parisienne in cream sauce—15 to 20	454	37	424	9	22	193	73
Gnocchi Parmigiana—12 to 16	425	28	1,090	19	24	114	59
Potato Gnocchi—12 to 16	264	8	751	12	37	85	27
Lasagne with ground beef—4 1/2" x 3 1/4" piece	811	55	565	29	40	129	61
Manicotti—10 oz. or 2 rolls	250	3	675	16	40	56	11
Ravioli, cheese filling, no sauce—5 oz.	310	4	140	16	53	40	12
Risotto with parmesan—12 oz.	745	37	1,519	16	86	42	45
Polenta with sausage—2" sq.	156	6	636	6	19	16	35
Polenta with cheese, sun-dried tomatoes, and olives—2" sq.	329	24	1,271	6	25	11	66

	Calories	Fat	Sodium	Protein	Carbos	Cholesterol	% Calories
		(g)	(mg)	(g)	(g)	(mg)	from Fat
Tortellini, cheese— 3/4 c.	260	6 g	290 mg	11 g	41 g	35 mg	21%
Tortellini, Sausage and pepper—3/4 c.	260	8	290	11	37	65	28
Ziti, baked, stuffed, vegetarian—slightly less than 3 oz. pasta with 2–3 oz. ricotta and 2/3 c. marinara sauce	750	40	523	31	66	142	48
MEAT							
Beef Braciole in tomato sauce—6 oz. meat	520	38	868	37	7	92	66
Calf Brains, fried—1 serving = 1/4 whole brain	294	20	1,384	15	13	1,858	61
Meatballs—1/4 lb. meat	387	27	321	23	13	187	63
Veal and Peppers— 12 oz.	964	66	325	72	21	272	61
Veal Scaloppini— 1/4 lb. veal							
with lemon sauce	287	17	185	25	8	117	53
with marsala	332	17	436	25	10	112	46
Veal shanks— *Ossobuco Milanese,* 1 serving = 1/2 lb. veal plus vegetables and broth	471	24	544	50	12	198	46
Veal Parmigiana— 1/4 lb. veal	1,201	90	1,067	49	50	198	67
Vitello Tonnato— (veal with tuna and egg) 1/3 lb. veal	847	77	519	36	4	177	82
Sausage, Italian— 1 link	160	13	365	6	5	35	73

	Calories	Fat	Sodium	Protein	Carbos	Cholesterol	% Calories
		(g)	(mg)	(g)	(g)	(mg)	from Fat
Carpaccio—3 oz. raw beef (Often served with 2 oz. parmesan and 1 T. olive oil)	179	9 g	54 mg	24 g	0 g	71 mg	43%
Prosciutto—1 oz. or 2 thin slices	65	4	524	8	0	23	55
Pepperoni—16 slices	130	12	530	6	0	30	83

FISH

Where nutritional values appear for steamed and broiled fish, add values if necessary for sauces and condiments from this and other menus.

	Calories	Fat	Sodium	Protein	Carbos	Cholesterol	% Calories
Anchovies in olive oil, drained—1 strip	8	<1	146	1	0	3	43
Calamari con vino—1/4 lb. squid	236	11	68	24	6	353	42
Caviar, black or red—1 T.	40	3	240	4	<1	94	68
Clams, steamed—20 small	133	2	101	23	5	60	12
Cod fish steak steamed with aioli sauce and vegetables (potatoes, carrots, artichoke), 1 serving = 8 oz.	668	44	297	35	35	126	59
Eel, broiled—3 oz.	200	13	55	20	0	137	59
Mussels in white wine and butter—1qt. mussels = 14 oz. = 18–20 mussels	190	11	341	14	7	56	52
Oysters, raw—6	58	2	94	6	3	46	33
Oysters, breaded and fried—6	173	11	367	8	10	71	57

	Calories	Fat	Sodium	Protein	Carbos	Cholesterol	% Calories
		(g)	(mg)	(g)	(g)	(mg)	from Fat
Red Snapper with sauteed vegetables—4 oz. fish (Whole fish is about 1 1/2 lbs.)	427	17 g	972 mg	40 g	30 g	63 mg	36%
Sardines, in oil—2	50	3	121	6	0	34	54
Scallops, breaded and fried—2 lg. scallops	67	4	144	6	3	19	47
Scampi—1/4 lb. shrimp	454	38	183	25	3	186	73
Zuppa di Pesce (seafood stew)—2 shrimp, 4 scallops, 1 1/2 oz. fish, and 2 mussels	187	5	707	24	10	95	24
CHICKEN							
Chicken, roasted with rosemary, skin on—1/4 chicken	362	24	103	34	1	113	60
Chicken Cacciatore—1/2 lb. meat	546	35	839	45	11	173	58
Chicken Parmigiana—1/4 lb. chicken breast	966	62	1,068	51	50	175	58
Chicken, Tuscan-Style with herbs, olives, raisins, and a light tomato broth; skin on—1/2 chicken	716	48	1,600	52	18	203	11
DESSERT							
Biscotti, hazelnut—1	50	2	32	1	7	17	36
Cheesecake, Italian 1/6 of a 9" pie	607	30	253	27	60	291	44
Figs—3	110	<1	2	1	29	0	4
Fruit Ice—1/2 c.	124	0	0	<1	31	0	0

	Calories	Fat	Sodium	Protein	Carbos	Cholesterol	% Calories
		(g)	(mg)	(g)	(g)	(mg)	from Fat
Macaroons—2 med.	180	9 g	13 mg	2 g	25 g	41 mg	45%
Sorbet—1/2 c.	135	2	44	1	29	7	13
Tiramusu—2 x 2 1/2" square	425	28	90	8	32	238	59
Zabaglione—2 T.	103	3	7	2	11	142	26
NUTS							
Almonds—1 oz.	167	15	3	6	6	0	81
Pine Nuts—1 oz.	146	14	1	7	4	0	86
Pistachio—1 oz.	164	14	2	6	7	0	77
GELATO							
Granita di Caffe con Panne—1/2 c.	155	15	17	1	6	54	87
Gelato di Caffe—1/2 c.	300	20	50	5	26	205	60
Gelato di Limone—1/2 c.	260	11	12	<1	42	41	38

34

FRENCH MENUS

FRENCH MENU SAVVY

Classic French dishes come with super-rich sauces, but the advent of nouvelle cuisine has lightened the fare. In place of butter, cream, and pork fat, exotic herbs, greens, and seasonings now provide flavor and texture. Not all small portions of artistically arranged food are low-cal, however. Our analyses of some of the recipes of the leading new-style chefs revealed that their preparations can be as calorie-intensive as the old-style dishes. There's a famous chicken salad from Ma Maison that torpedoes a diet with almost 600 calories and 41 fat grams in a serving. And Wolfgang Puck's salmon topped with a souffléed fish force has more than 35 grams of fat in a 3-ounce serving. With those statistics you might as well go for pork roast Normandy, with 48 fat grams, or a Swiss cheese soufflé with a mere 15 grams per serving.

Healthful menu choices are indicated by words such as poached, en brochette, fruit-based sauces, roast, grilled, steamed, wine and herbs, in foil or en papilliote, puree (usually, but ask).

Fat-filled choices are indicated by the words puff pastry, mousse, pâté, crème, au gratin, cheese or fromage, en croute, au beurre, hollandaise, béchamel, bordelaise, béarnaise, Mornay, mayonnaise.

Rules to Remember

• Don't be intimidated by even the fanciest French restaurant. You are the customer and the chef works for you.

- Despite rule number one, if you have strict dietary concerns, the best approach is to call ahead and discuss the menu. That gives the kitchen time to make a meal you want, and that they are proud of.
- Limit yourself to three courses per meal. It's so easy to fall for an appetizer, salad, a main course, vegetables, *and* dessert.

Sample FRENCH DINNERS for Every Appetite

	CALORIES	FAT
❖ **High-calorie meals**		
Ratatouille (1/4 c.)	192	14
Mixed field greens (1 1/2 c.)	33	<1
Vinaigrette dressing (1 T.)	92	10
Duck breast in wine, no skin (4 oz. meat)	285	7
French green beans (1/2 c., steamed)	111	<1
Red wine (6 oz.)	131	0

TOTAL CALORIES: 844
Fat grams: 32

	CALORIES	FAT
Potato leek soup (1 c.)	117	3
Mixed greens with 1 T. vinaigrette	112	10
Braised endive (1 endive)	84	8
Boeuf Bourguignon (8 oz. meat)	789	61
Chocolate mousse	348	23

TOTAL CALORIES: 1,450
Fat grams: 105

	CALORIES	FAT
Coq au vin (1/4 chicken)	706	55
French beans (1/2 c., with 2 tsp. butter)	177	7
Almond torte (1/10 of a 9" pie)	401	26

TOTAL CALORIES: 1,284
Fat grams: 88

	CALORIES	FAT
❖ **Medium-calorie meals**		
Escargot (6 snails with butter garlic sauce)	263	24
Mixed greens with 1 T. vinaigrette	112	10
Souffle, swiss cheese (1/6 of souffle)	210	15

TOTAL CALORIES: 585
Fat grams: 49

	CALORIES	FAT
Lobster à l'Américaine (1/2 of a 11/2 lb. lobster)	338	19
Asparagus (5–7 thin stalks, lemon juice, no butter)	35	<1
Raspberry sorbet (1/2 c.)	80	0

TOTAL CALORIES: 453
Fat grams: 19

	CALORIES	FAT
Soft-shell crabs (2, no egg batter)	486	33
Mixed greens with 1 T. vinaigrette	112	10

TOTAL CALORIES: 598
Fat grams: 43

❖ **Low-calorie meals**

	CALORIES	FAT
Cheese fondue (8–10 pieces of bread cubes and vegetables with 4–5 T. dip)	255	16
Tossed salad (1 T. oil and vinegar)	103	8

TOTAL CALORIES: 358
Fat grams: 24

	CALORIES	FAT
French bread (1 slice)	102	1
Salad Niçoise (lunch serving)	187	10
Peaches with raspberry sauce	153	<1

TOTAL CALORIES: 442
Fat grams: 11

	CALORIES	FAT
Onion soup (1 c. without cheese and bread)	155	9
Coquilles St. Jacques (3 oz. scallops)	143	7
Grilled zucchini (1 small)	118	11

TOTAL CALORIES: 416
Fat grams: 27

FRENCH MENUS

	Calories	Fat	Sodium	Protein	Carbos	Cholesterol	% Calories
		(g)	(mg)	(g)	(g)	(mg)	from Fat
BREADS							
Brioche—1 roll	286	17 g	443 mg	7 g	27 g	120 mg	53%
Croissant—1 roll	188	12	100	3	17	33	57
French bread—1 slice	102	1	203	3	19	0	9
Sourdough bread—1 slice	70	1	140	3	12	0	13
APPETIZERS							
Artichokes à la Grecque—3 sm. artichokes	334	15	**1,293**	12	39	0	40
Escargot à la Bourguignonne—6 snails in garlic butter	263	24	280	11	2	94	82
Olives, black—1 oz., or 4–5 med. olives	32	3	247	<1	2	0	84
Olives, green—1 oz., or 4–5 med. olives	33	4	680	<1	<1	0	100
Olive Tapenade—1 T.	44	4	163	1	1	0	82
Pâtés and Terrines: **Country-style Pâté**—1 slice about 2/3" thick	652	65	722	10	2	153	90
Duck terrine* with hazelnuts—1/24 of an 8-cup terrine, or about 2.5 oz.	509	50	369	8	3	107	89

*This recipe calls for duck livers and duck meat. Since data on duck liver are not available, data for 6 chicken livers were substituted for the 2 duck livers.

	Calories	Fat	Sodium	Protein	Carbos	Cholesterol	% Calories
		(g)	(mg)	(g)	(g)	(mg)	from Fat
Pâté de Volaille— (chicken pâté with pork) 1 slice, 1" thick	454	33 g	734 mg	31 g	3 g	165 mg	65%
Ratatouille—1/4 c.	192	14	290	3	16	0	66
Quiche:							
Lorraine—1/6 of 10" pie	914	80	1,064	14	34	309	78
Cheese—1/6 of 10" pie	499	34	836	14	33	211	61
SOUP							
Leek and Potato— 1 c.	117	3	840	2	19	13	23
Lobster Bisque—1 c.	350	28	559	12	9	112	72
Onion Soup—1 c. Without cheese and bread—(see separate listings if needed.)	155	9	1,256	4	15	16	57
Mushroom Soup with Cream—1 c.	483	48	971	6	11	170	89
Soupe au Pistou— 1 c.	375	21	2,515	11	39	5	50
Vichyssoise—1 c.	186	11	1,809	3	20	41	53
VEGETABLES							
Endive, braised— 1 endive	84	8	86	1	4	21	86
French Beans, steamed—1/2 c.,	111	<1	5	6	21	0	6
Petit Pois (green peas), steamed— 1/2 c.	67	<1	2	4	13	0	3

	Calories	Fat	Sodium	Protein	Carbos	Cholesterol	% Calories
		(g)	(mg)	(g)	(g)	(mg)	from Fat
Mushrooms							
Cèpes Paysanne—6 oz. fresh, 3 large or 6 small	128	7 g	385 mg	7 g	13 g	8 mg	49%
Champignons Cevenols, fresh, baked with garlic, parsley, olive oil, and breadcrumbs—4 oz.	276	28	154	3	7	<1	91
Chanterelles, fresh, cooked in chicken broth with shallots, chives, and butter—2 oz.	97	9	127	2	4	23	84
Creamed Button Mushrooms cooked with heavy cream, shallots, and herbs—6 lg.	481	45	46	6	17	153	84
Enoki, fresh, sauteed with soy, lemon, butter, and chives. (data approx.)—3.5 oz.	82	6	519	3	6	16	66
Oyster Mushrooms, no sauce or oil— 1 1/4 oz.	29	1	48	3	1	27	31
Potatoes							
Pommes Frites (french fries)— 20–25 1/2" strips	235	12	124	3	29	0	46
Puree de Pommes de Terre—6 oz.	335	20	281	6	35	59	51
Lyonnaise—3 oz.	155	9	555	2	18	22	52
Gratin Dauphinois—6 oz.	562	44	356	10	34	158	70
Potatoes Anna— 4 oz.	225	15	163	3	20	41	6

40

	Calories	Fat	Sodium	Protein	Carbos	Cholesterol	% Calories
		(g)	(mg)	(g)	(g)	(mg)	from Fat
Potatoes au Gratin with sausage—4 oz.	606	45 g	923 mg	19 g	31 g	281 mg	67%

SALADS

Mixed greens, no dressing—4 oz.	20	<1	10	1	4	0	14
Chicken Salad, made with egg, green beans, apple, tomato, mustard, mayonaisse and lemon juice— 1 c. on lettuce	589	41	521	41	15	237	63
Salade Niçoise— with 1 oz. canned tuna, 1/2 egg, 2 pieces anchovy, and dressing	187	10	846	18	6	127	48
Avocado–Fresh Tuna Salad—with 4 oz. tuna, egg, avocado, tomato, celery, cucumber, anchovy, and dressing	434	31	324	24	15	102	64

SALAD DRESSING

Roquefort—1 T.	77	8	167	<1	1	3	94
Vinaigrette—1 T.	92	10	55	<1	<1	0	98

OMELETTES

Cheese (Boursin)— 2 eggs	277	24	464	14	2	575	78

SOUFFLÉS

Salmon soufflé— 3 oz. filet of salmon, topped with seafood soufflé, for appetizer	429	35	574	25	2	135	73

41

	Calories	Fat (g)	Sodium (mg)	Protein (g)	Carbos (g)	Cholesterol (mg)	% Calories from Fat
Soufflé Démoulé, Mousseline, with Swiss cheese—1/6 soufflé	210	15 g	392 mg	12 g	6 g	146 mg	64%
Dessert Soufflés							
Soufflé au Grand Marnier—3/4 c.	295	14	226	11	30	241	48
Chocolate Soufflé—1/6 soufflé	414	21g	193	10	51	204	46
CRÊPES							
Crêpe, unfilled—1	141	6	162	5	16	84	38
Crêpe with Caviar and Sour Cream—1 crêpe	192	10	404	9	17	180	47
Crêpe with Shrimp and a Wine-Cheese Sauce—1 crêpe	346	24	324	12	20	180	62
Gâteau de Crêpes Florentine, with cheese, cream, and spinach—1/6 of a 24-layer stack of crêpes and sauces	1,009	62	1,194	35	77	487	55
Dessert Crêpes							
Apple—1 crêpe	279	17	198	5	27	119	55
Almond-brandy—1 crêpe	180	9	42	2	16	55	45
Fines Sucrées, with sugar and liquor—1 crêpe	92	4	39	2	10	45	39
Gâteau de Crêpes—1/6 of a 12-layered stack of crêpes, apples, and macaroons	415	18	162	5	60	113	39
Suzette—1	122	5	39	2	13	46	37

	Calories	Fat	Sodium	Protein	Carbos	Cholesterol	% Calories
		(g)	(mg)	(g)	(g)	(mg)	from Fat
Crêpe Topping, *Beurre d'Orange* (orange, liquor, sugar, and butter)—1 T.	44	4 g	<1 g	<1 g	2 g	10 mg	82%

SAUCES

	Calories	Fat	Sodium	Protein	Carbos	Cholesterol	% Calories
Au Jus—2 T.	5	<1	15	<1	<1	<1	0
Crème Anglaise—1 T.	27	1	7	<1	3	28	33
Crème Chantilly—1 T.	29	3	3	<1	<1	10	93
Béarnaise—1 T.	72	8	40	<1	<1	41	100
Béchamel—1 T.	31	2	14	<1	2	7	58
Bordelaise—1 T.	41	4	26	<1	<1	4	77
Gremolata (lemon, parsley, garlic sauce for fresh oysters)—1 T.	4	0	1	<1	<1	0	0
Hollandaise—1 T.	80	9	47	<1	<1	48	100
Mayonnaise—1 T.	112	13	28	<1	<1	16	100
Mignonette (spicy tomato tarragon for dipping fresh oysters)—1 T.	4	<1	69	<1	1	0	0
Mornay—1 T.	31	2	25	1	1	15	2

POULTRY

	Calories	Fat	Sodium	Protein	Carbos	Cholesterol	% Calories
Chicken Livers, sautéed, *Foies de Volaille*—3 oz.	338	17	283	22	18	522	45
Coq au Vin—1/4 chicken	706	55	1,012	39	13	169	70
Duck Breast with Port—4 oz. skinless meat	285	7	94	22	27	87	22

	Calories	Fat	Sodium	Protein	Carbos	Cholesterol	% Calories
		(g)	(mg)	(g)	(g)	(mg)	from Fat
Duck a l'Orange— 1/2 lg. duck with skin	1,599	123 g	668 mg	84 g	28 g	362 mg	69%
Goose, roasted—3 oz.	260	19	59	21	0	77	66
Pheasant, roasted— 1/4 of a bird, barded heavily with bacon and pork fat.	835	54	371	81	2	n.a.	5
Quail, roasted—See Greek section.							

FISH AND SHELLFISH

	Calories	Fat	Sodium	Protein	Carbos	Cholesterol	% Calories
Bouillabaisse—3/4 pound of assorted fish and shellfish in shells with approximately 1 1/4 cup liquid	484	21	819	59	13	150	39
Caviar, red or black— 1 T.	40	3	240	4	<1	165	68
Coquilles Saint Jacques—3 oz. scallops	143	7	162	13	7	35	44
Frogs' Legs—6 legs	230	12	316	19	8	176	47
Lobster a L'Americaine—1/2 of a 1 1/2-lb. lobster	338	19	558	17	15	85	51
Mussels Mariniere—1 qt., or 35–40 mussels	190	11	341	14	7	56	52
Red Snapper with scallop mousse—4 oz. fish and 4 oz. scallops	1,212	95	372	61	11	443	70
Salmon, poached, cold—6 oz. with 2 T. mayonnaise-caviar sauce	440	29	721	40	5	217	59
Sea Bass—8 oz. filet with sorrel and a cream sauce	548	35	178	44	8	189	57

	Calories	Fat	Sodium	Protein	Carbos	Cholesterol	% Calories
		(g)	(mg)	(g)	(g)	(mg)	from Fat
Shrimp with Mustard Cream sauce, *Crevettes à la Moutarde*—6–8 med. shrimp.	533	49 g	257 mg	14 g	6 g	203 mg	83%
Soft-shell crabs, dipped in egg and breadcrumbs, sauteed in lemon, beurre blanc, capers—2	799	63	405	38	19	238	71
Soft-shell crabs, prepared with blanched almonds, no eggs, and less butter than above—2	469	33	684	35	9	218	63
Smoked Fish Mousse, made with salmon, sturgeon, and caviar—2 oz.	244	22	585	12	2	137	81
Trout en Papilliote— 5 oz. filet with vegetables	234	10	89	30	7	82	38
Trout Sauteed with Almonds—6 oz. fish	746	62	745	38	10	223	75
MEAT							
Boeuf Bourguignon—about 8 oz. beef	789	61	686	45	14	195	70
Beef Wellington—6 oz. beef, with pastry. Most restaurant orders serve two.	1,572	124	1,892	48	69	320	71
Carbonnade de Boeuf—about 8 oz. beef	883	55	1,506	49	47	171	56
Cassoulet—3/4 c. beans with approximately 10 oz. of chicken, sausage, pork, duck and assorted vegetables	1,112	71	1,489	53	66	157	57

	Calories	Fat (g)	Sodium (mg)	Protein (g)	Carbos (g)	Cholesterol (mg)	% Calories from Fat
Cervelles au Beurre Noir, (beef brain in black butter)—5 oz. (1 whole brain is approximately 16 oz.)	519	45 g	598 mg	17 g	12 g	2,613 mg	78%
Filet Mignon—8 oz.	479	23	143	64	0	191	43
Pork Roast Normandy, with cream-mushroom sauce—4 to 5 oz. meat	688	48	99	40	15	209	63
Rabbit, roasted, no sauce—3 oz.	131	5	31	19	0	54	34
Rack of Lamb — 4 chops	732	58	843	41	9	185	71
Steak au Poivre— 10 oz. sirloin	780	55	294	55	6	213	63
Sweetbreads, *Ris de Veau,* braised— 5 to 6 oz.	242	12	354	28	3	426	45
Veal Kidney en Casserole, *Rognons de Veau*	595	33	1,084	63	8	1,500	50
Veal Loin, stuffed, with light sauce—5 to 6 oz.	764	43	470	67	12	771	51
Veal Orloff—about 8 oz. veal	993	70	1,000	63	28	355	63
Veal Stew—about 8 oz. veal	603	34	668	51	26	257	51
DESSERT							
Almond Torte—1/10 of 9" torte	401	26	54	9	35	176	58
Chocolate Mousse— 1 serving	348	23	69	8	36	127	59
Crème Caramel— 1 serving	263	6	82	7	46	153	21

	Calories	Fat	Sodium	Protein	Carbos	Cholesterol	% Calories
		(g)	(mg)	(g)	(g)	(mg)	from Fat
Eclair, with custard filling and chocolate icing—1 piece, about 5" x 2" x 1 3/4"	262	16 g	337 mg	6 g	24 g	127 mg	55%
Lady Fingers—1	40	<1	8	<1	7	39	19
Orange Sherbet—1/2 c.	135	2	44	1	29	7	13
Peaches with Raspberry Sauce—1 peach	153	<1	2	1	39	0	2
Pear Tart* with 2 oz. caramel sauce and 1 oz. whipped cream—1 med. slice	1,701	117	1,517	14	122	487	62
Raspberry Sorbet—1/2 c.	80	0	8	0	20	0	0
Sachertorte—1/10 of 9" torte	880	52	214	14	104	312	53
Sponge Cake—One 2 oz. slice	164	2	138	2	35	58	8
CHEESE AND DAIRY							
Brie—1 oz. (Double and triple creams are even more fat, calorie, and cholesterol laden.)	110	9	180	59	2	30	74
Camembert— 1 oz.	85	7	239	6	<1	20	74
Fondue—1 T. Swiss and Gruyère. (One dip of a cube of bread picks up about 1/2 T. of cheese.)	41	3	85	2	3	32	66
Gruyère—1 oz.	117	9	95	8	<1	31	69

* We found one chef who is so generous with his servings that his pear tart came to a whopping 2,268 calories per serving!

	Calories	Fat	Sodium	Protein	Carbos	Cholesterol	% Calories
		(g)	(mg)	(g)	(g)	(mg)	from Fat
Neufchâtel[1]—1 oz.	73	6 g	112 mg	3 g	<1 g	21 mg	74%
Port du Salut—1 oz.	98	8	150	7	<1	34	73
Roquefort—1 oz.	104	9	512	6	<1	26	78
Swiss, imported—1 oz.	100	7	155	7	1	25	63
Heavy Cream[2]—1 T.	52	6	6	<1	<1	20	95
Crème Fraîche—1 T.	52	6	7	<1	<1	20	98
Crème Fraîche, sweetened—1 T.	55	6	7	<1	1	20	98

[1]This is a light cream cheese. Regular cream cheese has around 100 calories an ounce and 10 grams of fat.

[2]This is whipping cream. In contrast, light cream has about 30 calories per tablespoon and 3 grams of fat. Half and half has 20 calories a tablespoon and 1.75 grams of fat.

MEXICAN AND TEX-MEX MENUS

MEXICAN AND TEX-MEX MENU SAVVY

Mexican and Southwestern foods can be healthful and delicious, but many restaurants pile on cheese, and sour cream, use lard in cooking, and serve portions that would sink an Armada. As a rule, you do best in non–fast-food Mexican and Tex-Mex restaurants where you have choices of grilled fish and meat and salads without cheese, guacamole, or fried taco shells.

True Mexican cuisine, like many styles of cooking around the world, does not depend on meat protein for its substance. Most meals feature no more than 2 or 3 ounces of meat. We'd do well to copy them and rely on rice, beans, and vegetables for the bulk of our calories. The smartest way to control cholesterol consumption is to avoid foods cooked with lard—common in refried beans and some meat dishes.

Salsa is pure goodness and can be heaped on food in place of cheese or guacamole—but don't heap it on taco chips. Without even noticing it, you can eat 20–30 chips before a meal. That adds up to 300 calories and 16 grams of fat—and you haven't even ordered yet!

Healthful foods are indicated by words such as grilled (fajitas), simmered, shredded, minced, soft tortilla, enchilada sauce, salsa.

Fat and cholesterol are indicated by words such as deep-fried, cheese, guacamole, nachos (any kind), huevos (eggs), buñuelos (fritters).

Rules to Remember

- Avoid all foods cooked with lard.
- Ask for combination plates, enchiladas, tacos and tostados without cheese, sour cream, or guacamole.
- Salsa is your friend. You can put it on anything and everything for great flavor without calories or fat.

Sample MEXICAN AND TEX-MEX DINNERS for Every Appetite

	CALORIES	FAT
❖ High-calorie meals		
Salsa with tortilla chips (1/4 c. with 12 tortilla chips)	175	10
Chicken fajita, without guacamole or sour cream (2 tortilla rolls)	514	20
Refried beans made with corn oil (1/4 c.)	120	5

TOTAL CALORIES: 784
Fat grams: 35

Guacamole (1/2 avocado)	218	20
Chips (12–14)	150	8
Beef burrito	680	32

TOTAL CALORIES: 1,048
Fat grams: 60

Enchiladas Suizas (2 tortilla rolls)	678	47
Refried beans, made with lard (1/4 c.)	120	5
White rice (1/2 c.)	176	<1
Sour cream (2 T.)	60	6

TOTAL CALORIES: 1,034
Fat grams: 58

❖ Medium-calorie meals		
Tamales, with pork and enchilada sauce (2)	410	28
White rice (1/4 c.)	88	<1
Tossed salad, 1 T. oil and vinegar	103	8

TOTAL CALORIES: 601
Fat grams: 36

	CALORIES	FAT
Ensalada de nopalitos (cactus salad)	60	4
Quesadilla with cheese and sour cream	513	36

TOTAL CALORIES: 573
Fat grams: 40

	CALORIES	FAT
Black bean chili (1 1/4 c.)	351	14
2 T. grated cheese	110	n.a.
Jalapeño cornbread	140	n.a.
1 beer	150	0

TOTAL CALORIES: 797
Fat grams: 23

❖ **Low-calorie meals**

	CALORIES	FAT
Grilled swordfish with salsa (1/2 order or 4 oz.)	200	5
White rice (1/4 c.)	88	<1
Ensalada de nopalitos (1 serving cactus salad)	60	11

TOTAL CALORIES: 348
Fat grams: 9

	CALORIES	FAT
Black bean soup (1 c.)	215	7
Chips (12–14 corn chips)	150	8
Salsa (1/4 c.)	25	2

TOTAL CALORIES: 390
Fat Grams: 17

	CALORIES	FAT
Cheese enchilada with enchilada salsa	333	22
White rice (1/4 c.)	88	<1

TOTAL CALORIES: 421
Fat grams: 22

MEXICAN/TEX-MEX MENUS

	Calories	Fat (g)	Sodium (mg)	Protein (g)	Carbos (g)	Cholesterol (mg)	% Calories from Fat
APPETIZERS							
Bean Dip—1/4 c.	228	14 g	182 mg	10 g	17 g	41 mg	55%
Chile con Queso—1/4 c.	152	12	336	7	5	39	71
Tortillas							
Chips—corn, 12–14	150	8	105	2	17	0	48
Corn—One 8" tortilla, made with corn oil	56	<1	40	1	12	0	10
Flour—One 8" tortilla, made with lard	162	9	92	2	18	8	50
Empanadas de Picadillo (ground meat turnover)—1	162	12	108	4	9	24	66
Guacamole—1 lg. avocado, plus seasonings	435	39	**1,147**	6	26	0	81
Jalapeños, stuffed with crabmeat—1 piece	136	9	146	11	3	88	60
Jalapeño Cornbread—1 piece 2" x 4"	140	5	240	3	22	20	32
Mexican Shrimp Cocktail—6 med. shrimp with avocado	205	15	260	12	9	96	66
Quesadillas, made with 2 6" tortillas, cheese, and sour cream—1	513	36	518	19	29	98	63
Wings and Drums—1 wing and 1 drum	273	18	640	24	3	76	59

	Calories	Fat	Sodium	Protein	Carbos	Cholesterol	% Calories
		(g)	(mg)	(g)	(g)	(mg)	from Fat
Nachos	**1,256**	**94 g**	**2,027 mg**	**54 g**	**54 g**	**213 mg**	**67%**
With Ground Beef—with 4 oz. beef, 3 oz. Monterey Jack cheese, olives, guacamole, sausage, refried beans, sour cream, salsa and onion							
Vegetarian—with 6 oz. cheddar cheese, peppers, tomatoes, spices, and 4 oz. tortilla chips	1,312	86	**2,155**	53	88	179	59
Salsa							
Enchiladas Salsa—1 T.	15	1	45	<1	2	<1	60
Green Salsa, Salsa Verde—1/2 c.	101	6	318	5	9	17	53
Pico de Gallo—1/2 c.	54	4	283	1	5	0	67
Red Salsa, Salsa Roja—1/2 c.	77	6	562	1	7	0	70
Salsa Fresca—1/2 c.	52	3	284	1	7	0	52
Watermelon Pico de Gallo—1/4 c.	14	<1	2	<1	3	0	6
CHILI							
Cubes of Beef, no beans—1 1/2 c.	504	16	1,715	58	39	132	29
Black Bean Chili—1–1 1/4 c.	351	14	1,204	20	39	32	36
REFRIED BEANS							
Black Beans with Bacon—1/2 c.	337	18	435	18	26	39	48

	Calories	Fat	Sodium	Protein	Carbos	Cholesterol	% Calories
		(g)	(mg)	(g)	(g)	(mg)	from Fat
Refried Pinto Beans with Corn Oil— 1/2 c.	240	9 g	5 mg	10 g	31 g	0 mg	34%
Refried Pinto Beans with Lard—1/2 c.	237	9	5	10	31	8	34
Refried Pinto Beans with Lard and Butter —1/2 c.	211	10	32	7	24	14	43
Note: If you stray from standard refried beans, chefs get fancy and calories add up!							

EGGS

	Calories	Fat	Sodium	Protein	Carbos	Cholesterol	% Calories
Huevos Rancheros— 2 eggs	569	42	601	17	31	425	66

SOUP

	Calories	Fat	Sodium	Protein	Carbos	Cholesterol	% Calories
Black Bean Soup— 1 c.	215	7	1,013	12	27	6	29
Sopa de Tortilla— 1 c.	171	9	335	7	21	0	47

SALAD

	Calories	Fat	Sodium	Protein	Carbos	Cholesterol	% Calories
Chicken Taco Salad—4 oz. tostada with 3 T. guacamole, 3 oz. chicken with beans, cheese, lettuce, tomatoes, pimento, green pepper and dressing	714	39	878	39	55	83m	49
Ensalada de nopalitos (cactus salad)— 1/2 c. nopales with garnish of onion, cilantro, tomato, feta cheese and dressing	60	4	269	3	4	13m	60

	Calories	Fat	Sodium	Protein	Carbos	Cholesterol	% Calories
		(g)	(mg)	(g)	(g)	(mg)	from Fat
CHICKEN							
Chimichanga—1 lg. tortilla roll	925	61 g	993 mg	38 g	57 g	91 mg	59%
Enchiladas Suizas— 2 tortilla rolls	678	47	787	32	33	93	62
Enchiladas Verdes con Pollo, (chicken enchilada with green salsa)—2 rolls	979	69	981	56	35	187	63
Fajitas, with chicken, onions, spices—for two tortillas	514	20	420	34	44	68	35
Add Salsa and 1/2 c. Guacamole to chicken fajitas above	905	51	871	40	75	68	51
Mole Poblano— 1/4 chicken	800	57	203	52	20	198	64
Pollo en salsa Chipotle (baked chicken with hot salsa)— 1/4 chicken, skin on	569	30	1,539	56	20	163	47
BEEF							
Burrito—one 12" tortilla	680	32	879	33	64	84	42
Picadillo, with beef and pork—(often used for empanada filling) 6 T.	445	37	352	21	8	89	75
Steak Fajitas—2 tortillas, 6 oz. beef, salsa, cheese, onions, green peppers, and guacamole	1,192	79	1,403	55	69	119	60
Taco—1 tortilla with ground beef, avocado, onions, salsa and spices	406	29	261	16	23	64	64

55

	Calories	Fat	Sodium	Protein	Carbos	Cholesterol	% Calories
		(g)	(mg)	(g)	(g)	(mg)	from Fat
Tamales, beef, with enchilada salsa— 1 tamale	253	19 g	295 mg	7 g	14 g	31 mg	68%
PORK							
Carne Adobado— about 6 oz. pork	475	35	567	33	6	132	66
Carnitas a la Casera—1/2 c.	253	18	347	20	1	81	64
Chiles Rellenos—3 green chiles filled with pork, tomatoes, and seasonings	809	59	**2,128**	35	37	265	66
Tamales*, Pork, with enchilada sauce— 1 tamale	205	14	225	7	13	29	61
Tostadas, with Carnitas a la Casera, refried beans, sour cream, guacamole and salsa—1	408	27	618	19	24	62	60
VEGETARIAN							
Chiles Rellenos with Cheese—1green chili	223	13	406	11	16	126	52
Enchilada, Cheese and enchilada salsa— 1 tortilla roll	333	22	557	14	26	43	59
Tamales*, Cheese and Hot Pepper— 1 tamale	174	12	234	4	12	19	62
Mexican Rice—1 c.	504	12	134	14	90	0	21

*One plain tamale made with lard has 8 mg cholesterol, while one made with vegetable shortening has 0 mg. Otherwise the fat, calorie, and sodium content are about the same. Adding meat or chicken increases all totals.

	Calories	Fat	Sodium	Protein	Carbos	Cholesterol	% Calories
		(g)	(mg)	(g)	(g)	(mg)	from Fat
FISH							
Ceviche—4 oz. scallops	427	15 g	465 mg	37 g	45 g	88 mg	32%
Red Snapper Vera Cruz—whole 2-lb. snapper	1,449	46	**5,929**	214	36	508	29
Swordfish, grilled, with salsa—8 oz.	395	9	215	43	38	79	21
Shrimp with ancho chile sauce—6 large shrimp	481	48	492	20	5	233	90
DESSERT							
Bread Pudding with Tequila Sauce—3" x 3" square with 1 T. sauce	673	3	473	9	87	177	41
Chile Custard—1/2–3/4 c.	576	49	225	7	29	376	77
Flan—5 oz.	316	9	142	10	50	202	26
Kahlua Mousse—1/2 c.	141	8	19	1	14	22	51
Kahlua Pie—1/6 pie	548	37	202	8	47	210	61
Sopapillas—1	282	19	530	2	26	0	61

SPANISH MENUS

SPANISH MENU SAVVY

Much Spanish food is similar to Provençal and Italian cooking, but the Mediterranean influence also brings a touch of North Africa into the kitchen. The result is an exceptional cuisine that offers vivid flavors and a wide selection of healthful fish and vegetable dishes, which are featured in the accompanying charts. (For information on various meat dishes, refer to the French, Italian, or Middle Eastern charts for similar recipes.)

Healthful foods are indicated by the words roasted, broiled, steamed, grilled, stewed.

Higher-calorie choices are indicated by the words creamed, fried, and breaded. Spanish-style pastas, lasagne, and other baked and cheesy pastas are as rich as Italian versions.

Rules to Remember

• Those scrumptious bite-sized appetizers can add up. Pay attention to what you choose and how many you eat.

Sample SPANISH DINNERS for Every Appetite

	CALORIES	FAT
❖ **High-calorie meals**		
Garlic soup (1 c.)	165	6
Grilled vegetables (mixed side dish)	187	11

	CALORIES	FAT
Codfish with tomato and red pepper sauce (4 oz. fish)	466	10

TOTAL CALORIES: 818
Fat grams: 27

	CALORIES	FAT
Paella Barcelona-style	620	27
Red wine (6 oz.)	144	0

TOTAL CALORIES: 764
Fat grams: 27

	CALORIES	FAT
Chicken in sherry sauce (1/4 chicken with 4–6 T. sauce)	826	56
Grilled vegetables	187	11
Tortilla Española (1/6 of a 10" pie)	352	23

TOTAL CALORIES: 1,365
Fat grams: 90

❖ Medium-calorie meals

Tapas:

	CALORIES	FAT
Bacon-wrapped dates (2)	82	3
Egg stuffed with anchovies and garlic (2 halves)	172	15
Eggplant mousse (3 T.)	78	6
Bread with tomatoes (1 slice)	96	4
Mushrooms stuffed with sausage (1)	76	5

TOTAL CALORIES: 504
Fat grams: 33

	CALORIES	FAT
Gazpacho rojo (3/4 c.)	200	15
Orange and avocado salad	299	27

TOTAL CALORIES: 499
Fat grams: 42

	CALORIES	FAT
Salt cod with potatoes and garlic	439	22
Green salad, with 1 T. vinaigrette	112	10

TOTAL CALORIES: 551
Fat grams: 32

	CALORIES	FAT

❖ Low-calorie meals

	CALORIES	FAT
Gazpacho rojo (3/4 c.)	200	15
Green salad, with 1 T. vinaigrette	112	10

TOTAL CALORIES: 312
Fat grams: 25

Saffron rice (1/2 c.)	209	6
Grilled vegetables	187	11

TOTAL CALORIES: 396
Fat grams: 17

Garlic soup (1 c.)	165	6
Bread with tomatoes (1 slice)	96	4
Eggplant mousse (1/4 c.)	104	8

TOTAL CALORIES: 365
Fat grams: 18

SPANISH MENUS

	Calories	Fat (g)	Sodium (mg)	Protein (g)	Carbos (g)	Cholesterol (mg)	% Calories from Fat
SAUCES							
Garum (Roman anchovy, olive dip)—1 T.	76	8 g	284 mg	<1 g	<1 g	14 mg	95%
Romesco Sauce with ancho chiles, onion, and paprika—1 T.	43	4	38	<1	2	<1	84
Salbitxada (Romesco-style sauce for grilled vegetables)—1 T.	51	5	22	<1	1	0	88
Salsa Roja (Romesco-style sauce for grilled fish)—1 T.	46	4	39	<1	1	0	78
Xato (Romesco-style sauce for Catalan Tuna Salad, *Xatonada*)—1 T.	56	6	28	1	<1	0	96
TAPAS							
Bacon-wrapped Dates, *Escolantets*—1 date	41	2	34	1	6	2	33
Bread with Tomatoes, *Pa amb Tomaquet*—1 slice peasant bread	96	4	143	2	14	0	38
Eggs Stuffed with Anchovies and Garlic, *Ou Farcits amb Anxova*—1/2 egg, stuffed	86	8	199	4	<1	83	78
Eggplant Mousse, *Mousse de Escalivada* or *Escum d'Escalivada* (grilled eggplant, pepper and tomato dip)—1 T.	26	2	70	<1	1	15	69
Mushroom Caps Stuffed with Sausage, *Xampinyons Farcits amb Xorico*—1 mushroom	76	5	269	3	4	7.5	59

	Calories	Fat	Sodium	Protein	Carbos	Cholesterol	% Calories
		(g)	(mg)	(g)	(g)	(mg)	from Fat
Prosciutto Croquettes, *Croquettes de Pernil*—1 croquette	43	3 g	116 mg	2 g	2 g	30 mg	63%
Salt-Cod Fritters, *Bunyols de Bacalla*—1" fritter	61	3	n.a.	6	2	33	44

SOUP

Garlic Soup with Thyme, *Sopa d'All i Farigola*—1 c.	165	6	**1,380**	5	18	<1	33
Gazpacho Rojo (red gazpacho)—3/4 c.	200	15	308	3	18	0	68

VEGETABLES

Grilled Mediterranean Vegetables, *Escalivada* —this recipe has a serving with 1/2 tomato, 4 strips eggplant, 4 strips red bell pepper, 1/2 onion; however, you can use the data as a guideline for most any mixture.	187	11	297	4	23	0	53
Leek Tart—1/8 of a 10" pie	518	38	426	12	36	194	66
Tortilla Española— (potato omelet served as Tapas or side dish) This serving contains 1 egg and is about 1/6 of a 10" skillet. If served as a main dish, triple the data.	352	23	347	9	28	213	59

SALAD

Orange and Avocado Salad—1/3 avocado, 1/3 orange with dressing	299	27	120	3	17	0	81

	Calories	Fat	Sodium	Protein	Carbos	Cholesterol	% Calories
		(g)	(mg)	(g)	(g)	(mg)	from Fat
Shredded Salt Cod Salad, *Esqueixada*—lunch-size serving with 2 to 3 oz. salt cod and dressing	516	33 g	n.a.	50 g	6 g	186 mg	58%
Tuna Salad with Xatonada, with escarole, anchovy, egg, olives, and Xatonada sauce—first course or lunch-size serving	509	45	802	17	12	87	80

RICE

Saffron Rice—1/2 c.	209	6	705	4	33	16	26
Rice with Raisins and Pine Nuts—2/3 c. rice	271	7	774	5	48	10	23
Paella Valenciana, classic version, with snails—1 c. rice, and sauce and 3 oz. chicken, 1 lg. prawn, 2 sm. meatballs, squid, 2 mussels, 1 clam, and 3 snails	954	38	1,068	69	82	372	36
Paella Barcelona-Style, *Arroz Barcelones,* made with pork, chorizo, pancetta, vegetables and grated cheese—1 c. rice with meat, sauce, and 1 oz. cheese	620	27	1,438	23	69	55	39

FISH

Codfish with Tomato and Red Pepper Sauce, *Bacalao Ajoarriero*—4 oz. cod	466	10	n.a.	74	17	173	19
Monkfish with Walnut Cream Sauce, *Rape con Nueces*—1/2 lb. fish	760	52	686	41	21	100	62

	Calories	Fat (g)	Sodium (mg)	Protein (g)	Carbos (g)	Cholesterol (mg)	% Calories from Fat
Fish Stew with Potatoes, Costa Brava–style, *Suquet de Pescado*—1 1/4 to 1 1/2 c. stew with about 5 oz. red snapper or other white fish	583	32 g	662 mg	36 g	26 g	56 mg	49%
Salt Cod with Potatoes and Garlic, *Brandada de Bacalla*—1/2 c. of mixture and a slice of bread fried in olive oil. (Sometimes this classic is made of nothing but cod, garlic, and cream. This is a milder, less caloric version.)	439	22	n.a.	42	17	120	45

CHICKEN

	Calories	Fat	Sodium	Protein	Carbos	Cholesterol	% Calories from Fat
Arroz con Pollo—3/4 c. rice with bacon and pork sausage and 8 oz. chicken	1,044	70	982	54	47	204	60
Chicken Samfaina with eggplant, zucchini, tomatoes and olives, *Pollastre amb Samfaina*—1/4 lg. chicken (Samfaina is sometimes served alone; here, it is used as a sauce.)	1,011	55	1,712	84	29	254	49
Chicken in Sherry Sauce, *Pollito de Grano al Vino de Jerez*—1/4 chicken with 4 to 6 T. cream-sherry sauce	826	56	842	57	13	263	61

DESSERT

	Calories	Fat	Sodium	Protein	Carbos	Cholesterol	% Calories from Fat
Musician's Tart, *Tarta de Musico*—1/8 of a 10" pie (This is a fancy version of Postre de Music, a mixture of dried fruits and nuts.)	597	26	144	9	81	92	39

JAPANESE MENUS

JAPANESE MENU SAVVY

Japanese food is one of the most healthful cuisines in the world—with a few notable exceptions.

The sodium level of many dishes could send the salt-sensitive, or those with high blood pressure, over the top.

The fried foods—tempura and fried dumplings in particular—are no better for you than fried food from Peking or Peoria.

And those little packages of delicious sushi, so light, so fat-free, can add up! If you're having two maki rolls and four pieces of sushi, for example, you may be surprised to know that you've taken in 1,000 calories. Add some fried dumpling appetizers and a beer, and you're taking in as many calories as if you stopped at a Mexican restaurant. The major difference is that you'll probably have eaten much less fat and cholesterol.

Healthful menu choices are indicated by words such as broiled, grilled, sushi, sashimi, steamed, soup.

Potential menu problems are indicated by the words fried (tempura) and—for those who watch their sodium intake—teriyaki, soy sauce, tamari, dipping sauce. In addition, remember that shellfish have relatively high cholesterol contents, and eel and fish roe are fatty.

Rules to Remember

• If you're concerned about eating raw fish, remember there are many alternative sushi choices:

Grilled eel, cooked shrimp, cooked crabmeat, smoked salmon, grilled salmon skin, vegetable makis, and various types of roe.

Sample JAPANESE DINNERS for Every Appetite

	CALORIES	FAT
❖ **High-calorie meals**		
Miso soup (1 c.)	97	2
Sea bass sashimi (4 oz.)	120	2
Yellowtail teriyaki (8 oz.)	422	6
Spinach with sesame dressing	76	5

TOTAL CALORIES: 715
Fat grams: 15

Yosenabe	680	24
Beer (12 oz.)	150	0

TOTAL CALORIES: 830
Fat grams: 24

California roll	327	16
Eel sushi (2 pieces)	180	6
Tuna maki	353	3
Salmon roe sushi (1 piece)	69	2
Sake (3 oz.)	72	0

TOTAL CALORIES: 1,001
Fat grams: 27

❖ **Medium-calorie meals**		
Sushi:		
2 pieces tuna	152	2
2 pieces mackerel	186	8
1 piece grilled eel	55	3
Boston roll (shrimp lettuce maki)	158	<1

TOTAL CALORIES: 551
Fat grams: 14

	CALORIES	FAT
Shrimp tempura (4 pieces)	291	8
White rice (1 c.)	265	<1
Spinach with sesame dressing (side dish)	76	5

TOTAL CALORIES: 632
Fat grams: 13

	CALORIES	FAT
Soba noodles (1/2 serving with soy-ginger sauce)	182	<1
Filet of sole (deep-fried)	321	11
Mixed salad with 2 T. Japanese dressing	148	14

TOTAL CALORIES: 651
Fat grams: 25

❖ **Low-calorie meals**

	CALORIES	FAT
Vegetable tempura (6 pieces)	308	9
Rice, white (1/4 c.)	66	<1

TOTAL CALORIES: 374
Fat grams: 9

	CALORIES	FAT
Sea bass sashimi	120	2
Brown rice (1 c.)	216	2
Spinach with sesame dressing	76	5

TOTAL CALORIES: 412
Fat grams: 9

	CALORIES	FAT
Chicken teriyaki (6 oz.)	364	6
White rice (1/4 c.)	66	<1
Mixed salad with lemon and soy dressing, no oil	25	<1

TOTAL CALORIES: 477
Fat grams: 6

JAPANESE MENUS

	Calories	Fat (g)	Sodium (mg)	Protein (g)	Carbos (g)	Cholesterol (mg)	% Calories from Fat
BASICS							
Soup, Miso—1 c.	98	2 g	755 mg	6 g	13 g	0 mg	18%
Rice, Brown—1 c.	216	2	4	5	45	0	8
Rice, Sushi—3/4 c.	265	<1	859	4	60	0	1
Rice, White, short grain—1 c.	265	<1	0	6	57	0	1
Salad Dressing, Japanese style oil and vinegar with soy sauce, sesame oil, ginger,—1 T.	64	7	22	<1	<1	0	98
Noodles, Soba, with soy, ginger, wahsabi dressing—3 oz.	363	<1	6,723	24	72	0	2
Noodles, Udon, 1/4 lb.	381	<1	899	16	85	0	2
Dipping Sauce—1 T.	10	<1	208	2	1	4	<1
Soy Sauce—1 T.	10	<1	1,029	<1	2	0	<1
Tamari—1 T.	11	<1	1,005	2	1	0	<1
SUSHI AND SASHIMI							
Maki							
California Roll, with crab meat and avocado—whole roll (usually cut into 6 pieces)	327	16	716	8	42	4	44
Boston Roll, with shrimp and lettuce—1 whole roll	158	<1	487	6	32	24	3

	Calories	Fat	Sodium	Protein	Carbos	Cholesterol	% Calories
		(g)	(mg)	(g)	(g)	(mg)	from Fat
Futomaki, with crab, cucumber, squash, egg—1 lg. roll	593	17 g	**2,427 mg**	32 g	77 g	486 mg	26%
Tuna Maki—1 roll	353	3	914	18	61	22	8
Sashimi*							
Sea Bass Sashimi with 1 tsp. dipping sauce—4 oz.	120	2	285	22	<1	50	15
Tuna Sashimi with 1 tsp. dipping sauce—4 oz., or six 3/4" cubes	184	6	264	28	3	47	29
Sushi							
Rice in Seaweed Wrap, without fish—1 piece	35	<1	116	<1	8	0	1
Fish to add to basic Sushi recipe above:							
Clam—1 piece	11	<1	8	2	<1	5	11
Crabmeat—1 oz.	29	<1	79	6	0	28	15
Eel, grilled with 1/2 tsp. sauce—1 oz.	55	3	129	5	<1	36	49
Egg Custard—1 oz.	33	2	22	2	3	30	41
Flounder—1 oz.	26	<1	23	5	0	14	11
Mackerel—1 oz.	58	4	26	5	0	20	62

*Serving sizes vary enormously. Small sashimi provides between 1 and 2 oz. very thinly sliced fish. (Use fish data under sushi for nutritional information.)

For special presentations you can double that amount. Sea bass and tuna, given here, represent the typical special dishes.

	Calories	Fat (g)	Sodium (mg)	Protein (g)	Carbos (g)	Cholesterol (mg)	% Calories from Fat
Fish Roe— 1 1/2 T.	34	2 g	0 mg	5 g	<1 g	90 mg	40%
Shrimp—1 piece	6	<1	9	1	<1	9	15
Squid—1/2 oz.	13	<1	6	2	<1	33	13
Tuna—1 oz.	41	1	11	7	0	11	22

FISH

	Calories	Fat (g)	Sodium (mg)	Protein (g)	Carbos (g)	Cholesterol (mg)	% Calories from Fat
Mizutaki (seafood and vegetable hot pot.) 1 large bowl with 1 c. rice, tofu, shrimp, scallops and vegetables	551	4	3,062	47	83	108	7
Salmon Teriyaki—8 oz. fish	500	18	1,546	47	21	125	32
Shrimp Tempura—4 pieces shrimp	291	8	680	25	26	193	25
Sole, Deep Fried, *Kareo kara Age—*6 oz. sole	321	11	n.a.	35	16	84	31
Tuna (Yellowtail) Teriyaki—8 oz.	422	6	1,530	55	21	102	13
Udon Suki—1 lg. bowl with 1/4 lb. udon noodles, 3/4 c. broth, and assorted vegetables, clams, shrimp, and chicken	645	5	4,098	53	102	172	13
Yosenabe—1 lg. bowl with 1 c. broth and assorted vegetables, clams, chicken, sea bass, mackerel, noodles, and tofu	680	24	2,655	75	33	252	32

CHICKEN

	Calories	Fat (g)	Sodium (mg)	Protein (g)	Carbos (g)	Cholesterol (mg)	% Calories from Fat
Teriyaki, Chicken—6 oz. breast	364	6	1,556	41	21	99	15

	Calories	Fat	Sodium	Protein	Carbos	Cholesterol	% Calories
		(g)	(mg)	(g)	(g)	(mg)	from Fat
Yakiitori, Chicken— 1 skewer with 2 oz. chicken and sauce (Sodium can double if sauce is not used sparingly.)	279	<1 g	1,760 mg	17 g	38 g	33 mg	3%
MEAT							
Rolled Beef with Asparagus—2 oz. beef per roll	177	12	224	11	4	38	61
Sukiyaki—6 oz. beef with rice noodles, tofu, spinach, and sauce	836	29	2,898	45	81	114	31
Teppanyaki (mixed grill with steak, prawns, scallops, and vegetables.)—2 oz. scallops, 1.5 oz. beef, and 2–3 shrimp	589	39	1,217	30	33	98	60
VEGETABLES							
Spinach with Sesame Dressing—2 oz. spinach in side-dish serving	76	5	377	3	7	0	59
Tempura, mixed vegetables—6 pieces	308	9	563	9	49	53	26

INDIAN, VIETNAMESE AND THAI MENUS

INDIAN, VIETNAMESE, AND THAI MENU SAVVY

Southeast Asian and Indian cuisines are basically healthful since they do not depend on meat for their main source of nutrition and dairy is scarce (except for ghee, the Indian clarified butter). They each rely on many grains and vegetables. They do present some challenges, however. Coconut milk and coconut meat are used in many soups and curries and both contain saturated fat. Fried food is common—Indian fritters, Vietnamese fried fish, and Thai fried noodles, for example.

Healthful foods on the menus are indicated by: stir-fried, steamed, soup (without coconut milk), simmered, tandoori, Tikka (grilled, skewered Indian dish), kebabs, biryani (without nuts), curried vegetables.

Higher fat foods are indicated by words such as crispy, fried, coconut, cream.

Rules to remember

• Avoid coconut products and fried foods and you can enjoy yourself without too much worry.

• Make meat a treat, not the main part of the meal.

Sample INDIAN DINNERS for Every Appetite

	CALORIES	FAT
❖ **High-calorie meals**		
Tomato chutney (4 T.)	76	4
Dal (3–4 oz. split peas)	177	7
Pakora (1)	96	5
Raita (1/4 c.)	33	2
Spiced lamb kabob (5–6 cubes of lamb)	412	19

TOTAL CALORIES: 794
Fat grams: 37

	CALORIES	FAT
❖ **Medium-calorie meals**		
Chapati (1)	122	2
Vegetable biryani (3/4 c. rice plus 3/4 c. vegetables)	360	11
Sweet mint chutney (4 T.)	52	<1

TOTAL CALORIES: 534
Fat grams: 13

	CALORIES	FAT
❖ **Low-calorie meals**		
Mixed vegetable curry (3/4 c.)	206	8
Basmati rice (1/2 c.)	100	<1
Mango chutney (2 T.)	42	<1

TOTAL CALORIES: 348
Fat grams: 8

INDIAN MENUS

	Calories	Fat (g)	Sodium (mg)	Protein (g)	Carbos (g)	Cholesterol (mg)	% Calories from Fat
BREADS							
Chapati—1 piece	122	2 g	139 mg	4 g	23 g	4 mg	15%
Rooti—1 piece	72	<1	172	3	15	<1	7
Dimer Parota (flaky bread with egg filling)—1 piece	245	10	202	7	33	73	37
Luchi (puffed bread)—1 piece 5" in diameter	120	6	61	2	14	0	45
CONDIMENTS and APPETIZERS							
Chutney Coconut—1 T.	29	2	7	<1	1	<1	62
Sweet Mint—1 T.	13	<1	2	<1	3	0	4
Tomato—1 T.	19	1	58	<1	2	0	47
Dal (lentils)—2 oz.	213	5	189	14	30	11	21
Dahl (split peas)—3–4 oz.	177	7	704	8	22	18	36
Ghee (the clarified butter used in many recipes)—1 T.	114	13	0	<1	0	33	100
Mulligatawny Soup—1 c.	152	5	499	10	18	8	30
Pakoras (mixed vegetable fritters)—1 fritter	96	5	122	3	10	0	47
Raita (yogurt cucumber dip)—1/2 c.	65	3	222	3	8	9	42
Rice, Basmati—3/4 c. cooked	150	<1	0	3	34	0	0

	Calories	Fat (g)	Sodium (mg)	Protein (g)	Carbos (g)	Cholesterol (mg)	% Calories from Fat
Samosas, (curried meat pastries)—1 piece	154	7 g	235 mg	6 g	16 g	21 mg	41%

MEAT AND CHICKEN

	Calories	Fat (g)	Sodium (mg)	Protein (g)	Carbos (g)	Cholesterol (mg)	% Calories from Fat
Spiced Lamb Kabobs—8 oz. (5–6 cubes) lamb	412	19	461	51	6	171	42
Tandoori Chicken—1/2 broiler	427	17	1,295	61	6	186	36
Chicken in Coconut Cream Sauce, *Murgi Malai Kari*—about six 1 oz. chunks of chicken	302	14	329	40	4	99	42
Skewered, Grilled Chicken, *Murgh Tikka*—6 oz. chicken marinated in yogurt	354	17	187	43	6	102	43

VEGETABLES

	Calories	Fat (g)	Sodium (mg)	Protein (g)	Carbos (g)	Cholesterol (mg)	% Calories from Fat
Biryani with vegetables—3/4 c. rice with 3/4 c. vegetables	360	11	329	8	58	17	28
Curried Cauliflower and Peas—1 c.	168	10	14	5	15	0	54
Eggplant in Cream Sauce—3/4 c.	233	12	24	6	30	4	46
Madras-Style Mixed Vegetables with Lentils—3/4 c.	180	6	19	8	25	0	30
Mixed Vegetable Curry—1 generous c., rice not included	274	12	790	8	38	32	39
Okra in Cumin and Garlic—1/2 lb. okra	199	10	23	6	24	0	45
Spicy Spinach—1/2 c.	179	11	221	8	17	0	55

Sample VIETNAMESE DINNERS for Every Appetite

	CALORIES	FAT
❖ High-calorie meals		
Lettuce roll with shrimp and meat (4)	184	5
Spring roll (1)	59	4
Vietnamese beef with ginger (4. oz beef)	375	26
Rice, white (1/2 c.)	133	<1

TOTAL CALORIES: 751
Fat grams: 35

	CALORIES	FAT
❖ Medium-calorie meals		
Asparagus crab soup (1 c.)	89	3
Spring roll (1)	59	4
Sea bass, steamed with vegetables and noodles (1/2 order, or 1 lb. fish)	350	10

TOTAL CALORIES: 498
Fat grams: 17

	CALORIES	FAT
❖ Low-calorie meals		
Chicken with mint leaves (3 oz.)	171	7
Rice paper (for wrapping chicken, 2 sheets)	112	2
Asparagus, steamed (8 thin stalks)	56	<1

TOTAL CALORIES: 339
Fat grams: 9

VIETNAMESE MENUS

	Calories	Fat (g)	Sodium (mg)	Protein (g)	Carbos (g)	Cholesterol (mg)	% Calories from Fat
SAUCES							
Nuoc Cham—1 T. (Used as commonly as salt and pepper, this sauce, can be very hot)	42	<1 g	<1 mg	1 g	8 g	0 mg	15%
Nuoc Leo—1 T. (used with meat dishes such as barbecued meatballs or beef with lemon grass and noodles)	24	2	9	<1	1	6	75
Buddhist Nuoc Leo—1 T. (used with vegetarian dishes and vegetarian spring rolls)	17	<1	<1	<1	2	0	39
Ginger Fish Sauce—1 T.	31	<1	1	1	5	0	21
APPETIZERS							
Asparagus Crab Soup, *Súp Măng Tây Cua*—1 c.	89	3	1,102	11	5	73	30
Beef Balls, *Bo Vien*—4 sm. balls, about 4 T.	239	11	330	29	4	72	41
Crab Fried with Salt, *Cua Rang Muoi*—1/2 lg. crab, or 2 crab claws (Salt can vary. Here, 1/4 tsp. per serving.)	105	8	540	8	1	39	69
Lettuce Rolls with Shrimp and Meat, *Cuon Diep*—2 packets	184	5	414	17	17	70	24
Rice Papers (Superthin crepes)—1 paper	56	1	<1	<1	10	0	16

	Calories	Fat (g)	Sodium (mg)	Protein (g)	Carbs (g)	Cholesterol (mg)	% Calories from Fat
Spring Rolls, with meat and fish filling—1 sm. roll	59	4 g	15 mg	2 g	4 g	17 mg	61%
Shrimp on Sugar Cane, *Chao Tom*—2 T. shrimp mixture on a 4" strip of sugar cane	338	17	114	15	29	97	45
ENTREES							
Beef Curry with coconut water and lemon grass, *Bo Kho*—4 oz.	354	18	1,818	31	16	62	46
Vietnamese Roast Beef with Ginger, *Be Thui*—4 oz. beef	375	26	57	21	12	81	62
Fried Chicken with Lemon Grass, *Ga Xao Sa Ot*—6 oz. chicken, or about 2 chicken thighs	455	23	156	49	11	160	45
Shredded Chicken with Mint Leaves, *Ga Xe Phay*—3 oz. meat	171	7	213	23	2	80	37
Vietnamese Chicken Curry, *Cari*—1/4 chicken	989	73	2,499	48	37	174	66
Fish, baked whole, stuffed with a noodle, vegetable, ground pork mixture, *Ca Rut Xuong Dut Lo*—whole 1 1/2-lb. sea bass	879	44	1,345	74	43	404	45
Fish, steamed with vegetables and noodles, *Ca Hap*—whole 2 lb. sea bass	700	20	879	83	44	185	26
Pork simmered with 5-spice powder, *Thit Thung*—4 oz.	406	28	676	22	15	81	62

Sample THAI DINNERS for Every Appetite

	CALORIES	FAT
❖ High-calorie meals		
Crispy fried snapper (4 oz.)	231	12
Thai fried rice (1/2 c.)	263	11
Stir-fried spinach with tofu (1 c.)	256	22

TOTAL CALORIES: 750
Fat grams: 45

	CALORIES	FAT
❖ Medium-calorie meals		
Thai beef salad (4 oz.)	559	34

TOTAL CALORIES: 559
Fat grams: 34

	CALORIES	FAT
❖ Low-calorie meals		
Spicy prawn salad (1/4 lb.)	168	3
Thai iced tea (10 oz.)	142	6

TOTAL CALORIES: 310
Fat grams: 9

THAI MENUS

	Calories	Fat (g)	Sodium (mg)	Protein (g)	Carbos (g)	Cholesterol (mg)	% Calories from Fat
FIRST COURSES and SIDE DISHES							
Hot and Sour Seafood Soup, *Tom Yum Talay*—1 1/2 c.	416	14 g	598 mg	55 g	15 g	229 mg	30%
Chicken in Coconut Soup, *Tom Kah Gai*—1 to 1 1/4 c.	461	31	384	32	15	66	61
Sticky Rice—3/4 c.	559	21	50	5	91	0	34
Sticky Rice with Mangoes—3/4 c. rice	627	22	52	6	108	0	32
Thai Fried Rice—1 c. rice with 2–3 oz. pork, crab, and shrimp	525	22	623	34	45	190	40
Thai Satay— (pork loin marinated in coconut milk and spices, served on skewers)—5oz.	339	15	308	46	3	143	40
Stir-fried Spinach—1 c., cooked with tofu, tomato, and spices	256	22	187	8	13	0	77
Crispy Fried Vermicelli, *Mee Krob*—2 oz. noodles with pork, chicken, shrimp, vegetables, and mushrooms (A restaurant portion often contains 2 servings.)	844	40	839	66	52	245	43
COLD COURSES							
Spicy Prawn Salad, *Yaam Goong*, 1/4 lb., or 8–9 med. shrimp	168	3	148	22	15	140	16

	Calories	Fat (g)	Sodium (mg)	Protein (g)	Carbos (g)	Cholesterol (mg)	% Calories from Fat
Thai Beef Salad— 4 oz. beef	559	34 g	624 mg	25 g	39 g	81 mg	55%
VEGETABLES							
Hot and Sour Stir-fried Vegetables, *Pad Pak Priew Waan*—2/3 c. mixed vegetables (may include green beans, carrots, cabbage, zucchini, onion) and spices	134	10	550	2	11	0	67
FISH							
Mussels steamed with spicy coconut-milk sauce—about 7 mussels	242	18	645	9	12	58	67
Shrimp with Lemon Grass—5 oz. shrimp	279	14	1,542	31	7	224	44
Sweet and Sour Shrimp—3 oz. shrimp	301	15	1,306	20	20	140	45
Red Snapper, crispy fried filets—4 oz. fish	231	12	74	24	7	42	47
MEAT							
Green Curry Beef— 4 oz. beef, not including rice	623	52	1,525	26	14	77	75
Ginger Beef, spicy, fried—4 oz. beef	390	31	62	23	4	76	72
Red Curry Pork— 4 oz. pork, not including rice	492	39	214	29	9	75	71

	Calories	Fat	Sodium	Protein	Carbos	Cholesterol	% Calories
		(g)	(mg)	(g)	(g)	(mg)	from Fat

CHICKEN

	Calories	Fat (g)	Sodium (mg)	Protein (g)	Carbos (g)	Cholesterol (mg)	% Calories from Fat
Chicken Curry, *Gaeng Pet Gai,* with coconut milk—4 oz. chicken breast and approx. 5 oz. sauce	480	37 g	643 mg	30 g	11 g	66 mg	69%
Chicken Masaman Curry, *Gaeng Daeng Gai,* with potatoes and peanuts—7 oz. chicken meat	720	48	607	47	28	164	60

DESSERT

	Calories	Fat (g)	Sodium (mg)	Protein (g)	Carbos (g)	Cholesterol (mg)	% Calories from Fat
Mango Ice Cream— 1 scoop	734	45	118	3	87	163	55
Thai Iced Tea— 1 glass	142	6	88	5	18	22	38
Mango Slices— 1/2 c.	66	<1	2	1	16	0	0
Stewed Bananas in Syrup, *Glouy Boud Chee*—1 plantain	412	15	38	4	76	0	32

CARIBBEAN AND AFRICAN MENUS...PLUS

CARIBBEAN MENU SAVVY

Caribbean restaurants are becoming popular in the United States, but many people first encounter the cuisine when they head to the islands for a vacation. One of the joys of Caribbean travel is that on each island (or group of islands) the cuisine has evolved from a unique blend of native foods, African heritage, and the cuisine of the colonial power that once dominated the area (St. Maarten's food has a Dutch influence; Martinique's is French; Barbados' is English). Wherever you visit, you'll find an abundance of healthful, tasty choices. And the same is true at a restaurant stateside.

Healthful menu items are indicated by words such as stew, curry (without coconut or coconut milk), poached, steamed, grilled.

High-fat items are indicated by words such as fried, coconut, peanut, cream, pudding, fritter.

Rules to Remember

- For lower-fat meals stick with grilled fresh fish.
- Remove the paper umbrella from your glass before you take a drink.

Sample CARIBBEAN DINNERS for Every Appetite

	CALORIES	FAT
❖ High-calorie meals		
Conch chowder (1 1/4 c.)	291	1
Peppery poached red snapper (1/2 whole snapper)	384	4
Green salad with 1 T. vinaigrette	112	10

TOTAL CALORIES: 787
Fat grams: 14

	CALORIES	FAT
Banana fritter (1 piece)	90	3
Crab stew (without coconut milk)	446	12
Mango mousse (1 c.)	209	4
Frozen Daiquiri (1 drink)	119	<1

TOTAL CALORIES: 864
Fat grams: 19

	CALORIES	FAT
Jerk chicken (1/2 chicken)	693	40
Beans and rice (4 oz. beans and 3/4 c.)	384	8
Green salad with 1 T. vinaigrette	112	10

TOTAL CALORIES: 1,189
Fat grams: 58

❖ Medium-calorie meals	CALORIES	FAT
Curried goat with vegetables (8 oz. meat)	372	13
White rice (1/2 c.)	132	<1

TOTAL CALORIES: 504
Fat grams: 13

	CALORIES	FAT
Banana fritters (two pieces)	180	6
Escovitched fish (1/4 lb.)	180	6
Bahamian rice and peas (1/2 c.)	215	9

TOTAL CALORIES: 575
Fat grams: 21

	CALORIES	FAT
Beefsteak Creole (1/2 order, or 4 oz.)	243	17
Fried green plantains (4 slices)	249	21
Green peas (1/2 c.)	67	<1

TOTAL CALORIES: 559
Fat grams: 38

	CALORIES	FAT
❖ **Low-calorie meals**		
Callaloo soup (1 1/2 c.)	302	10

TOTAL CALORIES: 302
Fat grams: 10

| Shrimp Curry (5 oz. shrimp with sauce, no coconut) | 284 | 11 |
| White rice (1/2 c.) | 132 | <1 |

TOTAL CALORIES: 416
Fat grams: 11

| Bahama Mama (1 drink) | 148 | 3 |
| Yellow Bird (1 drink) | 153 | <1 |

TOTAL CALORIES: 301
Fat grams: 3

CARIBBEAN MENUS...PLUS

	Calories	Fat (g)	Sodium (mg)	Protein (g)	Carbos (g)	Cholesterol (mg)	% Calories from Fat
SAUCES							
Creole Tomato Sauce, *Salsa Criolla Cocida* in the Dominican Republic—1 T.	37	3 g	1 mg	<1 g	2 g	0 mg	73%
Farofa de Dende Brazil's basic palm oil-based pepper sauce—1 T.	56	3	2	<1	6	0	48
Hot Pepper Sauce sometimes called crushed peppers—1 T.	12	<1	36	<1	3	0	15
Mango Chutney—1 T. This recipe is from Trinidad.	21	<1	2	<1	5	0	3
Mango Salsa—1 T.	7	<1	<1	<1	2	0	3
Papaya Chutney—1 T.	9	0	31	<1	2	0	0
Sauce Chien, sometimes *Sauce Chienne* a spicy French-Caribbean sauce served with seafood and poultry—1 T.	134	14	29	<1	3	0	94
SOUP							
Avocado Curry Soup—1 c.	281	27	1,003	3	11	41	86
Callaloo Soup— 1 1/2 c. Caribbean gumbo, called *Calalou* in the French Antilles, it's made with ham, beef, callaloo leaves or spinach, okra, potatoes, and spices. Crab meat is often added.	302	10	2,975	32	24	11	30

	Calories	Fat	Sodium	Protein	Carbos	Cholesterol	% Calories
		(g)	(mg)	(g)	(g)	(mg)	from Fat
Conch Chowder or Conch Soup—1 1/4 c.	291	1 g	294 mg	31 g	40 g	74 mg	3%
Pigeon Pea Soup— 1 c. Called *Gungo Peas* in Jamaica and Trinidad, *Gandules* or *Gandures* in Spanish-speaking islands	282	9	n.a.	20	31	31	29
Pumpkin Soup—1 c. A favorite on St. Lucia and other islands	432	25	2,050	38	13	82	52

APPETIZERS

Coconut Bread—1" slice. Favored on Grenada and other islands	271	15	168	5	31	30	50
Escovitched Fish, *Pescado en Escabeche* (Pickled snapper or mackerel) 1/2-lb. filet. Prepared the traditional way this is a low-fat treat. But see MAIN COURSE, where tweaked just a bit, it becomes much heavier a dish.	360	12	883	48	13	84	30
Feroce d'Avocat Spicy avocado spread—1 T.	50	4	n.a.	2	2	4	72
Accras de Moreu Salt cod fritters from Martinique and Guadeloupe—one 1 1/4" fritter	127	3	n.a.	15	8	45	21
Akkra on Jamaica; on Curacao called *Calas* (Black-eyed pea fritters)—one 1 1/4" fritter	70	2	3	3	9	0	26
Banana Fritters— about 1/4 banana	90	3	49	1	15	18	30

	Calories	Fat	Sodium	Protein	Carbos	Cholesterol	% Calories
		(g)	(mg)	(g)	(g)	(mg)	from Fat
Fried Green Plantain, Called *Banane Pese* on French Islands and *Tostones* on Spanish ones—4 slices of 3/4" wide strips	249	21 g	71 mg	<1 g	18 g	0 mg	76%
Jamaican Beef Patties, A spicy empanada with a beef mixture in a half-round pastry shell—1 piece 2 1/2" across	284	15	584	11	27	41	48
Puerto Rican Sofrito, made with salt pork, ham, tomatoes, and olives—1 T.	50	5	192	1	2	7	90
CHICKEN							
Arroz con Pollo— 1/4 chicken with 1 1/4 to 1 1/2 c. rice	1,091	50	686	54	94	174	41
Chicharrones de Pollo—fried chicken, on the Spanish islands—1/2 lg. boneless breast	550	26	249	49	25	130	43
Chicken in Coconut Milk, *Fricassee de Poulet au Coco* in Martinique, *Poulet a la Creole* in Haiti—1/2 lb. chicken	868	73	180	47	9	174	76
Jerk Chicken, Jamaica—1/2 chicken	693	40	1,662	70	14	220	52
Keshi Yena Coe Galinja (or *Keshy Yena* on the Dutch islands) Baked Edam stuffed with shredded spiced chicken—1/6 of a 4-lb. stuffed Edam	760	44	1677	70	21	216	52

	Calories	Fat (g)	Sodium (mg)	Protein (g)	Carbos (g)	Cholesterol (mg)	% Calories from Fat

FISH

	Calories	Fat (g)	Sodium (mg)	Protein (g)	Carbos (g)	Cholesterol (mg)	% Calories from Fat
Conch Stew—1/2 lb. conch, without rice (data an approximation)	412	11 g	471 mg	55 g	20 g	148 mg	24%
Crab Stew, *Matoutou de Crabes* on Martinique and Guadeloupe— about 5 oz. crab meat and 1 c. rice with sauce	446	12	374	31	51	132	24
Crab Pilau Tobago, Crab stew above, with curry powder, onion, and coconut milk—5 oz. crab meat and 1 c. rice with sauce	764	44	396	35	59	132	52
Escoveitche de Pescado*—8 oz. fish.	893	65	876	50	29	84	66
Fish Curry, *Colombo de Poisson* with 1/2-lb. shark filet. On the French islands this curry is made with lamb, chicken, and fish.	546	31	449	50	10	116	51
Jerk Red Snapper, Jamaica. 1/2-lb. filet	323	9	1,602	49	14	84	25
Peppery Poached Red Snapper, *Poisson en Blaff* on Martinique and Guadeloupe—1/2 whole red snapper	384	4	714	51	17	87	9
Plantains and Marinated Fish Filets—1/2 plantain and 5 oz. flounder, cod, or perch	421	12	447	38	38	174	26

*This illustrates how different chefs can change the content of any food. This marinated fish dish is similar to the appetizer given above, but it is pan-fried, marinated in a richer sauce, and served cold.

	Calories	Fat (g)	Sodium (mg)	Protein (g)	Carbos (g)	Cholesterol (mg)	% Calories from Fat
Salt Fish with Ackee, Jamaica's national dish—1/4 lb. dried salt cod	773	47 g	n.a.	76 g	10 g	197 mg	55%
Shrimp Curry—with 5 oz. shrimp and sauce, not including rice	284	11	596	28	19	207	35
MEAT							
Beefsteak Creole, *Biftek a la Creole* on Martinique—8 oz. steak	487	34	90	39	<1	131	63
Curried Goat, On French islands, *Colombo d'Agneau*—1/2 lb. meat (On Jamaica and other English islands this dish is sometimes made with mutton.)	372	13	742	49	15	129	31
Feijoada, Brazil's famous black bean and meat cassoulet— 1 1/2 c.	1,141	70	2,815	73	53	180	55
VEGETARIAN							
Bahamian Rice and Peas—1 c. rice with peas and vegetable sauce	431	18	366	7	58	16	38
Beans and Rice Cubano, *Habichuelas y Arroz Cubano,* with black turtle beans, 3/4 c. rice and 4 oz. beans	384	8	8	12	66	0	19

	Calories	Fat	Sodium	Protein	Carbos	Cholesterol	% Calories
		(g)	(mg)	(g)	(g)	(mg)	from Fat
DESSERTS							
Banana Pudding with Rum Sauce— 1 1/4 c.	415	16 g	221 mg	5 g	50 g	103 mg	35%
Bread Pudding with Brandy Sauce—about 1 1/4 c.	749	41	830	18	77	287	49
Coconut Custard from Guadeloupe—1/6 of 9" pie (On Spanish-speaking islands, *Tembleque* is similar.)	546	22	134	11	76	164	36
Ginger Mousse— 3/4 c.	326	11	166	12	34	172	30
Mango Mousse—1 c.	209	4	29	3	43	14	17
Rum Creme Surprise, a frozen dessert recipe from Jamaica found throughout the islands—1 scoop	311	11	55	6	39	140	32
DRINKS							
When you dine in the Caribbean, fancy drinks are often an integral part of the experience. Here's a look at what they contribute nutritionally.							
Bahama Mama— 1 drink	148	3	12	<1	19	0	18
Frozen Daiquiri— 1 drink	119	<1	5	<1	6	0	<1
Yellow Bird— 1 drink	153	<1	7	<1	11	0	<1
Rum Rickey— 1 drink	103	<1	30	<1	2	0	<1

AFRICAN MENU SAVVY

African restaurants are becoming more common in the U.S., particularly those featuring Ethiopian and Moroccan food. But most of us have been enjoying African cuisine for years without recognizing it. African cooking styles have had a huge impact on the cuisines of the southern U.S., the Caribbean, and South America—particularly in Brazil, Guyana, and Surinam. Many dishes that we think of as Brazilian, Caribbean, or Louisianan are virtually unchanged from their transatlantic cousins. According to Jessica Harris, author of a collection of Creole, Cajun, and Caribbean recipes called *Iron Pots and Wooden Spoons*, the Caribbean's Callaloo soup is almost identical to the African Soupikandia. Martinique's Matoutou Crabes is a culinary descendant of Benin's Ago Glain. And the Brazilian national dish, Feijoada, was brought to this hemisphere by practitioners of the West African religion Candomble: The bean and meat stew is the food associated with their god Ogun. In addition, the South's okra and gumbo dishes are of African origin.

This section features the nutritional information for a few typical dishes from Morocco, Ethiopia and other countries.

Healthful menu items are indicated by words such as stewed, roasted, grilled.

High-fat items: Although it is hard to make generalizations about cuisines from an area as vast and diverse as Africa one caveat does apply—Avoid palm kernel oil, a staple in many areas of the continent (and in Brazil); it is high in saturated fat.

AFRICAN MENUS

	Calories	Fat (g)	Sodium (mg)	Protein (g)	Carbos (g)	Cholesterol (mg)	% Calories from Fat
Many Caribbean and South American dishes are derived from African cuisines. Middle Eastern cuisine overlaps with North African cooking styles. Here are several classics from various parts of the continent.							
Berbere, hot spice mixture used in Ethiopian and Eritrean cooking—1 tsp.	3	<1 g	138 mg	<1 g	<1 g	0 mg	27%
Niter Kebbeh, spiced clarified butter from Ethiopia—1 T.	207	23	235	<1	<1	62	100
Peanut Sauce, appears in many African dishes—1 T.	19	1	41	<1	2	0	47
Couscous, Moroccan lamb and vegetable stew on couscous (pearls of semolina wheat) 1 1/2 c.	746	21	227	46	92	114	25
Fish Couscous, made with a firm white fish (here, striped mullet) and vegetables— 1 1/2 c.	682	6	553	37	120	39	7
Senegalese Seafood Stew *Thiebou Dienne.* The national dish of Senegal is often served as a one-pot meal from which everyone feasts. —1 1/2 c.	285	6	570	23	37	94	19

	Calories	Fat	Sodium	Protein	Carbos	Cholesterol	% Calories
		(g)	(mg)	(g)	(g)	(mg)	from Fat
Ethiopian Spicy Mixed Vegetable Stew, *Yetakelt W'et*—1 1/4 to 1 1/2 c.	316	24 g	995 mg	4 g	24 g	62 mg	68%
Gombo with tomatoes, based on a recipe from Benin—1/2 c. *Gombo* is the Swahili word for okra, which is featured in many African, Caribbean, and creole dishes.	89	4	563	3	13	0	40
Harira, the national soup of Morocco—1 c.	200	9	900	5	27	0	41
Vegetable Tajine (Moroccan stew)—1 1/2 c. without rice or couscous	249	14	823	4	29	0	50
Lamb Tajine with fruit and honey—5 oz. lamb	378	14	97	32	32	97	33

GREEK AND MIDDLE EASTERN MENUS

GREEK AND MIDDLE EASTERN MENU SAVVY

Greek and Middle Eastern cuisines have much in common, favoring lamb, aromatic herbs and spices, grilled and stuffed vegetables, and fresh vegetable salads of all types. As you peruse the menu at your favorite restaurant, keep an eye out for such specialties. Most are low in fat and calories and taste great. On a Greek menu the only potential trouble spots are in baked dishes such as moussaka or pastitsio. And on both Greek and Middle Eastern you want to take it easy on the tasty appetizer dips made from eggplant, chick peas, and tahini.

Rules to Remember

• Concentrate on vegetable and grain dishes to control fat and calories.

Sample GREEK AND MIDDLE EASTERN DINNERS for Every Appetite

	CALORIES	FAT
❖ High-calorie meals		
Eggplant dip (4 T.)	40	2
Pita bread (1/2 large home-style)	155	2
Lentil salad (1/2 c.)	180	8
Souvlakia marinated lamb skewer (three 1" cubes meat)	146	8

	CALORIES	FAT
Tzatziki (cucumber yogurt sauce) (4 T.)	58	2
Baklava (1/2 piece 2" x 1.5")	130	8

TOTAL CALORIES: 709
Fat grams: 30

	CALORIES	FAT
Stuffed grape leaves (3 rolls)	171	9
Moussaka (4 " square)	691	51
Rice pudding (1/2 cup)	246	7

TOTAL CALORIES: 1,108
Fat grams: 67

❖ **Medium-calorie meals**

	CALORIES	FAT
Fish Plaki (1/2 pound cod)	323	10
Salad with cucumbers and tomatoes	65	0
Oil and lemon dressing (2 T.)	140	10

TOTAL CALORIES: 528
Fat grams: 20

	CALORIES	FAT
Pita bread (1/2 large home-style)	155	2
Taboule (3/4 c.)	320	1
Squid salad (3 oz.)	220	15

TOTAL CALORIES: 695
Fat grams: 18

❖ **Low-calorie meals**

	CALORIES	FAT
Greek salad (1/2 large dinner-sized)	323	25

TOTAL CALORIES: 323
Fat grams: 25

	CALORIES	FAT
Avgolemono soup (3/4 c.)	64	3
Spinach pie (4" x 2 1/2")	235	18

TOTAL CALORIES: 299
Fat grams: 21

GREEK MENUS

	Calories	Fat	Sodium	Protein	Carbos	Cholesterol	% Calories
		(g)	(mg)	(g)	(g)	(mg)	from Fat
APPETIZERS							
Avgolemono Soup (lemon, egg, rice soup)—3/4 c.	64	3 g	762 mg	5 g	6 g	71 mg	42%
Eggplant Dip with yogurt and mayonnaise —1 T. (Sometimes called eggplant salad.)	10	<1	4	<1	2	<1	44
Feta Cheese, marinated—2 oz. (Plain feta has 60 calories per 2 oz.)	232	21	634	8	3	51	81
Iman Bayaldi (baked stuffed eggplant slices)—3–4 sm. slices	219	15	245	6	21	0	62
Pita Bread, large, thick, home-style—1 whole round	310	4	369	10	58	0	12
Spinach Pie, *Spanakopitta,*—4" x 2 1/2" piece	235	18	417	7	12	73	69
Stuffed Grape Leaves, *Dolmades,* stuffed with rice and seasonings—1 rolled grape leaf	57	3	69	1	6	0	47
Taramasalata—2 T.	180	14	n.a.	6	9	72	70
Tzatziki, yogurt cucumber sauce—2 T.	29	1	386	2	3	5	31
COLD DISHES							
Squid Salad—3 oz. squid, in average appetizer-sized serving. Main entree may be double.	220	15	43	14	6	206	61

	Calories	Fat (g)	Sodium (mg)	Protein (g)	Carbos (g)	Cholesterol (mg)	% Calories from Fat
Greek Salad with tomatoes, cucumbers, 6 olives, 3 oz. feta cheese, and dressing made with 2 T. oil and 1 T. lemon juice—dinner entree.	646	50 g	1,215 mg	20 g	38 g	76 mg	70%
Lentil Salad—1 c.	360	15	16	18	43	0	38
ENTREES							
Eggplant, Stuffed—1/2 eggplant with ground lamb, creamy tomato sauce, cheese	529	35	589	24	31	84	60
Fish Plaki—1/2 lb. fish filet (Data here for cod.)	323	10	293	43	16	98	28
Ground Meat Pastries, filo dough stuffed with ground beef and seasonings—one 3" roll, not including Tzatziki	133	10	177	6	5	21	68
Keftedes, fried meat patties—one 1 1/2" patty	86	6	36	5	3	24	63
Lamb Pastries, lamb in grape leaves and filo dough with seasoning—one pastry, 3 1/2" to 4" long, with 2 oz. lamb	359	30	295	11	11	62	75
Moussaka with ground lamb—4" square	691	51	521	28	28	122	66
Pastitsio—3 1/2" x 4" rectangle	729	45	896	35	45	121	56
Pork Kabob, marinated and served with tomatoes, onions, and green peppers—1 skewered, with three 1" cubes	164	11	38	11	4	45	60

	Calories	Fat	Sodium	Protein	Carbos	Cholesterol	% Calories
		(g)	(mg)	(g)	(g)	(mg)	from Fat
Quail, broiled with spices—2 quail	586	45 g	117 mg	43 g	2 g	n.a.	69%
Souvlakia, marinated lamb chunks —1 skewer, with three 1" cubes, not including Pita Bread or yogurt sauce	146	8	48	16	2	48	49
Swordfish Kabob, marinated and served with tomatoes and onions—skewered with three 1" cubes of fish	139	9	54	12	2	22	58
DESSERT							
Baklava—4" x 3" piece	259	15	112	4	28	25	52
Honey Cake—1 "cake" 2" in diameter	235	9	2	2	36	0	35
Kadaifi—1 roll 3" long	228	12	134	4	28	7	46
Rice Pudding, Rizogalo—1/2 c.	246	7	78	7	40	74	26

MIDDLE EASTERN MENUS

	Calories	Fat	Sodium	Protein	Carbos	Cholesterol	% Calories
		(g)	(mg)	(g)	(g)	(mg)	from Fat
As Caribbean and African cuisines overlap, so occasionally do North African, Middle Eastern, and Greek. Refer to those other sections for supplemental information.							
APPETIZERS							
Baba Ghanoush— 1 T.	13	1 g	20 mg	<1 g	1 g	0 mg	69%
Eggplant Puree for dipping—1/4 c. or 4 T.	47	5	1	<1	2	0	19
Falafel—three 2" patties	310	4	740	13	22	0	12
Hummus bi Tahini— 1 T.	57	3	7	2	6	0	5
Tahini Dip—1 T.	47	4	79	1	2	0	77
Taboule—3/4 c.	320	1	530	5	33	0	3
ENTREES							
Burghul Pilav with Lamb, a Turkish specialty made with cracked wheat, lamb, onions, and tomatoes— 1 1/2 c. with 1/4 lb. lamb	803	40	502	36	82	158	45
Kibbeh*, fried— 1 patty 2" in diameter	323	10	84	21	39	50	28

*The national dish of Lebanon and Syria, Kibbeh is a mash of lamb and cracked wheat eaten raw or cooked. Variations include sandwiches, stuffed rolls, or in Egypt rice and lamb.

	Calories	Fat (g)	Sodium (mg)	Protein (g)	Carbos (g)	Cholesterol (mg)	% Calories from Fat
Stuffed Vegetables*							
All Meat filling, *Sheikh* el Mahshi or *Tatbila*—1/4 c.	268	20 g	141 mg	20 g	6 g	75 mg	67%
Meat and rice filling—1/2 c. (This filling is the most common.)	177	4	48	13	20	37	20
Persian filling with meat, rice, and yellow split peas—1/2 c.	277	11	120	17	27	57	36
Vegetarian Rice filling, used for cold vegetables—1/2 c.	102	<1	7	2	22	0	2
Turkish filling for eggplant—Turkish filling with lamb, tomato, onion and cheese—1/2 c.	302	21	98	15	16	48	63

*Mahshi are favorites throughout the Middle East. Eggplant stuffed with rice, meat and spices is a classic favorite, although any vegetable can be used. The data given here is for the stuffing, where most of the calories come from. To figure out the nutritional information for a complete dish, refer to the Basic Foods section for vegetable data.

GERMAN, EASTERN EUROPEAN, AND SCANDINAVIAN MENUS

GERMAN, EASTERN EUROPEAN AND SCANDINAVIAN MENU SAVVY

Scandinavian, Eastern European, and German food is hearty, made to fight the cold and fuel the hard-working. However, neither we nor they have to fight the cold or do physical labor as much anymore. That means that the meaty stews, compact dumplings and cream-rich casseroles are a shortcut to a thick waist.

You can eat leaner if you stick to roasted meats—with sauces and gravy on the side—steamed vegetables, and fresh fruit. But if you want to enjoy classic *Eastern European* or *German* food the best bet is not to indulge too frequently, and when you do, close your eyes, open your mouth, and enjoy. *Scandinavian* cuisine offers more seafood choices.

Healthful cooking is indicated by the words steamed, boiled, roasted (no skin!), grilled.

Fatty food is indicated by the words sour cream, spiced, cream or creamed, dumplings, wurst, fried, breaded, cheese.

Rules to Remember

• Eat half orders of whatever shows up on your plate. That's the easiest way to control fat and calories since so many dishes depend on fatty meats and rich sauces.

• Make a meal out of simple vegetables and potatoes, with meat as an accent.

Sample GERMAN DINNERS for Every Appetite

	CALORIES	FAT
❖ High-calorie meal		
Potato pancake (1, with 1/4 c. applesauce)	270	14
Sauerkraut (1/2 c., plain)	25	0
Venison cutlet (6 oz., with mushroom sauce)	353	18
Pfeffernusse cookie (1)	150	2

TOTAL CALORIES: 798
Fat grams: 34

❖ Medium-calorie meal		
Venison cutlet (6 oz.)	353	18
Red cabbage with apples (5 oz.)	165	5
Beer (12 oz.)	146	0

TOTAL CALORIES: 664 (518 without beer)
Fat grams: 23

❖ Low-calorie meal		
Sauerkraut, plain steamed (1 c.)	50	0
Bratwurst (1)	341	29
Potato dumplings (2)	84	6

TOTAL CALORIES: 475
Fat grams: 35

GERMAN MENUS

	Calories	Fat (g)	Sodium (mg)	Protein (g)	Carbos (g)	Cholesterol (mg)	% Calories from Fat
DUMPLINGS and NOODLES							
Butter Dumplings, *Butterklosse,*—2 small dumplings	44	3 g	75 mg	2 g	3 g	41 mg	61%
Egg Noodles, 1 c. cooked, plain	200	2	3	7	37	50	9
Liver Dumplings, *Leberklosse,*—three 1 1/2" dumplings	251	14	806	19	11	433	50
Potato Dumplings, *Kartoffelklosse*—one 1" dumpling	42	3	116	<1	4	17	65
Spatzen, *Spatzle* or *German Egg Dumplings*—about 1/2 c.	438	26	628	9	41	168	53
VEGETABLES							
Potato Pancake—one 4" pancake, with 1/4 c. applesauce	270	14	379	4	33	65	47
Potato Salad, hot German-style—6 oz.	352	22	453	7	32	25	56
Red Cabbage with Apples—5 oz. cabbage	165	5	755	3	30	4	27
Sauerkraut,* plain— 1/2 c.	25	0	700	1	4	0	0
Sauerkraut,* steamed and spiced —1/2 lb. sauerkraut	388	21	2,702	25	22	67	49

*This data is for undrained and unrinsed sauerkraut. Prepared dishes are usually well drained and rinsed.

	Calories	Fat (g)	Sodium (mg)	Protein (g)	Carbos (g)	Cholesterol (mg)	% Calories from Fat
ENTREES							
Beef in spiced sour cream, *Wurzfleisch*—1/2 lb. beef	654	43 g	696 mg	52 g	11 g	173 mg	59%
Beef Goulash—5-plus oz. meat, or 5–8 chunks of beef; not including noodles	471	37	629	29	3	103	71
Beefsteak Tartare, with anchovy, egg, and capers—4 oz. beef	296	16	**7,468**	32	6	292	49
Chicken Paprika—1/2 breast or thigh, plus wing and drumstick	882	69	**1,304**	34	12	242	70
Rabbit, Braised, *Hasenpfeffer*—1 lb. meat	739	41	752	74	12	222	50
Rollmops, marinated herring—2 rolled herring filets	224	11	n.a.	21	12	66	44
Sauerbraten—1/2 lb. beef	828	61	154	43	26	209	66
Venison Cutlets, *Rehschnitzel mit Pilzen*—6 oz. cutlet with 3 T. mushroom-cream sauce	353	18	360	41	6	185	46
Weinerschnitzel, breaded veal cutlet—1/3 lb. veal	600	32	920	55	21	280	48
WURSTS							
Bratwurst—one 4 oz. link	341	29	632	16	2	68	77
Braunschweiger—2 oz.	204	18	648	8	2	88	79
Knockwurst—one 4 oz. link	349	31	**1,145**	13	2	66	80

	Calories	Fat (g)	Sodium (mg)	Protein (g)	Carbos (g)	Cholesterol (mg)	% Calories from Fat
DESSERT							
Apfelpfannkuchen, apple-filled pancakes— one 10" pancake	668	43 g	648 mg	14 g	59 g	**386 mg**	58%
Linzertorte—1/12 of a 9" torte, or a wedge that's 1 3/4" to 2" across at the widest part	302	17	179	4	36	66	51
Pfeffernusse—1 cookie	150	2	45	2	33	3	12
Sachertorte—1/12 of a 9" cake, or a wedge that's 2" across at the widest part	527	29	249	7	68	154	50
Strudel, Apple—3" x 3" square	296	9	142	4	52	35	27

Sample EASTERN EUROPEAN DINNERS for Every Appetite

	CALORIES	FAT
❖ **High-calorie meal**		
Beef Goulash (5 oz., or about 5 chunks, beef)	487	38
Egg noodles (2 oz.)	215	5
Red cabbage with apples (5 oz.)	165	5

TOTAL CALORIES: 867
Fat grams: 48

	CALORIES	FAT
❖ **Low-calorie Meal**		
Blintzes (2)	334	18
Sour cream (2 T.)	50	6
Applesauce (1/2 c.)	88	<1

TOTAL CALORIES: 472
Fat grams: 24

EASTERN EUROPEAN MENUS

	Calories	Fat	Sodium	Protein	Carbos	Cholesterol	% Calories
		(g)	(mg)	(g)	(g)	(mg)	from Fat
Food from Eastern Europe and foods associated with Jewish cuisine have become standard American fare. Here are some of the most popular.							
Beef Goulash— 5 oz. beef	487	38g	686mg	27g	7g	130mg	70%
Beef Stroganoff—8 oz. meat, not including noodles or rice	1,095	94	727	49	15	362	77
Blintzes, cheese-filled crepes—1 blintz	167	9	433	10	14	88	49
Borscht—1 c. broth-based beet soup with cabbage, beef and topped with 2 T. sour cream	175	12	769	10	7	48	62
Kasha Varnishkes, Russian for buckwheat, this dish is made by adding egg noodles, onions, and butter—3/4 c.	321	7	710	11	54	82	20
Potato Latkes—one 2 1/2" latke, plain	101	5	87	2	11	28	45
Ruggelach—1 pastry	81	5	16	1	10	12	56

Sample SCANDINAVIAN DINNERS for Every Appetite

	CALORIES	FAT
❖ **High-calorie meal**		
Lamb and cabbage casserole (6 oz. lamb)	527	41
Apple pudding (1/2 serving)	250	16

TOTAL CALORIES: 777
Fat grams: 57 (!)

	CALORIES	FAT
❖ **Medium-calorie meal**		
Cherry soup (3/4 c.)	289	16
Prawn salad open-face sandwich (2 sandwiches)	264	10

TOTAL CALORIES: 553
Fat Grams: 26

	CALORIES	FAT
❖ **Low-calorie meal**		
Gravad lox (2 oz.)	88	4
Dill sauce (2 T.)	168	18
Dark bread (2 thick slices)	220	3

TOTAL CALORIES: 476
Fat grams: 25

SCANDINAVIAN MENUS

	Calories	Fat	Sodium	Protein	Carbos	Cholesterol	% Calories
		(g)	(mg)	(g)	(g)	(mg)	from Fat
APPETIZERS							
Cherry Soup—3/4 c.	289	16 g	15 mg	2 g	30 g	54 mg	50%
Danish Liver Pate—1" slice	281	21	446	10	13	147	67
Danish open-faced sandwiches These favorites come in many variations. Bread can be rye, white or dark.							
Prawn Salad—5 med. shrimp, 1 slice bread, and lemon juice	132	5	240	8	13	66	34
Smoked Salmon and Egg—1 oz. salmon, 1 egg, and 1 slice of bread	243	15	499	14	13	240	56
Roast Beef and Potato —1 oz. thin- sliced beef, 2 oz. boiled potato, mayonnaise, and mustard	304	18	338	12	24	42	53
Cheese-Radish-Cucumber—1 oz. Swiss cheese with vegetables	210	13	249	10	14	37	56
Potato and Salami—2 oz. salami, with 2 oz. potato and 1 slice of on rye	403	24	**1,307**	17	28	55	54
Gravad Lox—2 oz., or 2 thick slices, or 6 thin ones (In the U.S. we often slice lox paper thin, but thick slices are traditional.)	88	4	n.a.	11	2	31	41

	Calories	Fat	Sodium	Protein	Carbos	Cholesterol	% Calories
		(g)	(mg)	(g)	(g)	(mg)	from Fat
Dill Sauce for Gravad Lox—1 T.	84	9 g	7 mg	<1 g	<1 g	0 mg	96%
Norwegian Fish Mousse—1/2 c.	203	15	515	10	7	97	67
Prawn Sauce for Mousse—1 T.	28	2	39	1	<1	17	64
ENTREES							
Jansson's Frestelse, an onion, potato, and anchovy casserole—1 c.	482	33	915	11	37	113	62
Norwegian Lamb and Cabbage Casserole—6 oz. lamb and 1/6 head of cabbage (If lamb is well trimmed the calories, etc. fall dramatically.)	527	41	503	33	6	136	70
Spiced Herring—1/4 lb. or 1 1/2 to 2 filets	249	11	668	22	14	74	40
Swedish Hash and Eggs, *Pytt i panna*—1 egg, fried with 1 1/4 c. hash	588	32	452	40	33	313	49
Swedish Meatballs—1 meatball about 1 1/2" in diameter	221	17	134	12	6	76	69
DESSERTS							
Danish Apple Pudding—1 c., topped with 3 T. whipped cream	502	32	409	3	56	84	57

	Calories	Fat	Sodium	Protein	Carbos	Cholesterol	% Calories
		(g)	(mg)	(g)	(g)	(mg)	from Fat
Red Fruit Pudding, a dessert variation of the common fruit soups with raspberries, red currants, and strawberries—1 c.	509	7 g	52 mg	4 g	101 g	0 mg	12%
Swedish Pancakes—three 3" pancakes and 1 T. jam	402	27	177	8	33	180	60

BASIC FOODS

This Basic Foods section is designed to help you make a rough estimate of the nutritional content of specific dishes not listed under the individual cuisines in this book. Refer to those sections for figures on sauces and seasonings. Add that information to the basic date given here. You should be able to get a pretty good picture of the calorie and fat content of almost any menu item.

	Calories	Fat (g)	Sodium (mg)	Protein (g)	Carbos (g)	Cholesterol (mg)	% Calories from Fat
FISH							
These basic fish data are for uncooked 8 oz. fillets.							
Catfish, wild—8 oz.	263	10 g	143 mg	41 g	0 g	132 mg	34%
Catfish, farm-raised—8 oz.	290	16	75	34	0	75	50
Clams—3 oz	65	1	102	11	2	43	14
Cod—8 oz.	186	2	122	40	0	98	10
Crab meat, canned—2 oz.	34	<1	335	23	1	135	14
Flounder—8 oz.	206	3	184	43	0	109	13
Halibut—8 oz.	249	5	122	47	0	73	18
Monkfish—8 oz.	172	3	41	33	0	57	16
Pompano—8 oz.	372	21	147	42	0	113	51
Salmon—8 oz. (average data)	322	14	100	45	0	125	39
Sea Bass—8 oz.	220	5	154	42	0	93	20
Snapper—8 oz.	227	3	145	47	0	84	12
Sole—8 oz.	206	3	184	43	0	1091	13
Swordfish—8 oz.	274	9	204	45	0	88	30
Tuna—8 oz.	327	10	88	53	0	86	33

	Calories	Fat (g)	Sodium (mg)	Protein (g)	Carbos (g)	Cholesterol (mg)	% Calories from Fat

MEAT

A menu tells you the weight of a steak before cooking, not the amount of meat you end up being served. For example, an 8-ounce T-bone yields only about 3 1/2 ounces of lean meat on your plate. Eight ounces of beef tenderloin or filet mignon ends up being about 7 1/2 ounces after cooking. Some meat data are given for what are called 8-ounce portions of meat, but they reflect the nutritional levels of edible meat actually served.

Beef

	Calories	Fat (g)	Sodium (mg)	Protein (g)	Carbos (g)	Cholesterol (mg)	% Calories from Fat
Ground, Lean— 3 oz.	230	16 g	65 mg	21 g	0 g	74 mg	63%
Ground, Extra Lean—8 oz.	430	27	118	43	0	141	57
Liver, fried— 3 oz.	185	7	90	23	7	**410**	34
Prime Rib, large— 4.6 oz. lean meat after cooking	329	19	96	36	0	107	52
T-bone, lean only—8 oz. (3.53 oz. edible)	214	10	66	28	0	80	42
Tenderloin, lean only—8 oz. (7 to 7.5 oz. served rare)	480	24	144	64	0	192	45
Veal, broiled— 3 oz.	185	9	56	23	0	109	44

	Calories	Fat (g)	Sodium (mg)	Protein (g)	Carbos (g)	Cholesterol (mg)	% Calories from Fat
Lamb							
Leg, Lean—2.6 oz.	140	6 g	50 mg	112 g	0 g	65 mg	39%
Pork							
Bacon—3 slices	110	9	303	6	<1	16	74
Chop, Lean, broiled—5 oz.	330	16	20	46	0	142	44
Ham, Lean, roasted—2.4 oz.	105	4	902	17	0	37	34
POULTRY							
Chicken with Skin, broiled—1/2 of a 2 1/2 lb. chicken	596	33	205	68	0	220	50
Chicken without Skin, broiled—1/2 of 2 1/2 lb. chicken (7.2 oz. chicken meat)	388	15	175	59	0	182	35
Turkey, Dark Meat, roasted—1 piece 2 1/2" x 1 5/8" x 1/4"	40	2	17	6	0	18	45
Turkey, Light Meat, roasted—1 piece 4" x 2" x 1/4"	67	2	26	13	0	28	27
VEGETABLES							
Artichoke, steamed—1 med.	60	<1	114	4	13	0	3
Asparagus, steamed—4 oz., about 4-5 thin stalks with the bottoms off	28	<1	5	3	5	0	11
Beans, green, steamed—1/2 c.	22	<1	2	1	5	0	7

	Calories	Fat (g)	Sodium (mg)	Protein (g)	Carbos (g)	Cholesterol (mg)	% Calorie from Fat
Beans, Baby Lima—1/2 c.	95	<1 g	26 mg	6 g	18 g	0 mg	5%
Beans, Snap—1/2 c.	23	<1	2	1	5	0	1
Bean Sprouts (Mung)—1/2 c. raw	15	<1	3	2	3	0	<1
Beets, cooked—1/2 c.	27	<1	43	1	6	0	<1
Black-eyed Peas—1/2 c.	90	<1	4	7	15	0	4
Broccoli, cooked—4 oz.	32	<1	29	3	6	0	<1
Brussels Sprouts—7–8 sprouts	60	1	33	4	13	0	15
Cabbage, Bok Choy—1 c.	20	<1	58	3	3	0	<1
Cabbage, Green—1 c.	20	<1	20	1	4	0	<1
Cabbage, Red—1 c.	20	<1	8	1	4	0	<1
Carrots, cooked—1/2 c.	35	<1	51	<1	8	0	4
Cauliflower, cooked—1 c. or 5 florets	30	<1	7	2	6	0	6
Collards, plain—1 c.	25	<1	36	2	5	0	<1
Corn on the Cob, boiled—1 sm. ear	77	1	14	3	17	0	12
Eggplant, Steamed—1 c.	25	<1	3	1	6	0	<1
Peas, steamed—1/2 c.	67	<1	2	4	13	0	2
Pickle, Dill—one 3"–4" long	5	<1	928	<1	1	0	<1
Pickle, Sweet—2 1/2" long	20	<1	107	<1	5	0	<1

	Calories	Fat	Sodium	Protein	Carbos	Cholesterol	% Calories
		(g)	(mg)	(g)	(g)	(mg)	from Fat
Potato, baked—6 oz.	124	<1 g	9 mg	3 g	29 g	0 mg	<1%
Potato Chips—10 chips	105	7	94	1	10	0	60
Potato, French Fried—10 fries	160	8	108	2	20	0	45
Spinach, steamed—1/2 c.	21	<1	63	3	3	0	10
Sweet Potato, baked—1 med.	115	<1	11	2	28	0	<1
Tomato, raw—one 2 1/2" diameter	26	<1	11	1	6	0	14
Zucchini, steamed—1/2 c.	14	<1	3	<1	4	0	3
FRUIT							
Apple—one 2 3/4" diameter	81	<1	0	<1	21	0	5
Applesauce—1 c. unsweetened	105	<1	5	<1	28	0	<1
Apricots—1/2 lb.	17	<1	<1	<1	4	0	7
Avocado, California—1	305	30	21	4	12	0	89
Banana—one 8 3/4" long	105	<1	1	1	27	0	5
Blackberries—1/2 c.	38	<1	9	1	20	0	12
Blueberries—1/4 lb.	64	<1	7	<1	16	0	6
Cantalope—1/2 med.	95	1	24	2	22	0	9
Cherries—10	50	1	<1	1	11	0	18
Dates, whole—2	46	<1	<1	<1	12	0	0
Grapes, Green—10	35	<1	1	<1	9	0	<1

	Calories	Fat	Sodium	Protein	Carbos	Cholesterol	% Calories
		(g)	(mg)	(g)	(g)	(mg)	from Fat
Grapefruit—1/2 of one 3 3/4" diameter	38	<1 g	0 mg	<1 g	10 g	0 mg	3%
Kiwi—1 med.	46	<1	4	<1	11	0	6
Mango—1 med.	135	<1	4	1	35	0	4
Orange—one 2 1/3" diameter	69	<1	0	1	17	0	4
Papaya—one-half of one large 5 1/2" high and 3 1/2" diameter	59	<1	5	<1	15	0	3
Peach— one 2 1" diameter	37	<1	0	<1	10	0	2
Pear, Bartlett—one 3 1/2 " tall and 2 1/2" diameter	98	<1	0	<1	25	0	6
Pineapple, fresh, chunks—1 c.	75	1	2	1	19	0	12
Plantains, cooked, plain—1 c.	180	<1	8	1	48	0	<1
Plum—one 2 1/8" diameter	36	<1	0	<1	9	0	10
Raspberries—1/4 lb.	56	<1	0	1	13	0	10
Strawberries—1/4 lb., or 6 med. berries	33	<1	1	<1	8	0	11

PIES

1/6 of average-sized home-style

	Calories	Fat	Sodium	Protein	Carbos	Cholesterol	% Calories
Apple	405	18	476	3	60	0	40
Blueberry	380	17	432	4	55	0	40
Custard	330	17	436	9	36	169	46
Lemon Meringue	355	14	395	5	53	143	35
Pecan	575	32	305	7	71	95	50

	Calories	Fat (g)	Sodium (mg)	Protein (g)	Carbos (g)	Cholesterol (mg)	% Calories from Fat
CANDIES AND SWEETS							
Caramel—1 oz.	115	3 g	64 mg	1 g	22 g	1 mg	23%
Chocolate, Milk—1 oz.	145	9	23	2	16	6	56
Chocolate, Semisweet—1 oz.	143	10	4	2	16	0	63
Chocolate Sauce—2 T.	85	<1	36	1	22	0	<1
Chocolate Fudge Sauce—2 T.	125	5	42	2	21	0	36
Jams and Preserves—1 T.	55	<1	2	<1	14	0	<1
Sugar, Granulated—1 T.	45	0	0	0	12	0	0
Syrup, Maple or Corn—2 T.	122	0	19	0	32	0	0
DAIRY AND EGGS							
Butter, salted—1 T.	100	11	116	<1	<1	31	99
Cheese, Cheddar—1 oz.	110	9	180	7	<1	30	74
Cheese, Swiss—1 oz.	110	9	50	8	1	25	74
Cream, Light—1 T.	30	3	6	<1	1	10	90
Cream, Half and Half—1 T.	20	2	6	<1	1	6	90
Cream, Heavy—1 T.	50	6	6	<1	<1	21	100
Cream, Sour—1 T.	30	3	7	<1	1	13	90
Egg—1 whole	75	5	63	6	1	213	60

	Calories	Fat (g)	Sodium (mg)	Protein (g)	Carbos (g)	Cholesterol (mg)	% Calories from Fat
Egg Yolk—1	60	5 g	7 mg	3 g	<1 g	213 mg	75%
Egg White—1	15	0	55	4	<1	0	0
OILS							
Corn—1 T.	125	14	0	0	0	0	100
Peanut—1 T.	125	14	0	0	0	0	100
Safflower—1 T.	125	14	0	0	0	0	100
BREADS							
Pumpernickle, flat, European style— 1 slice	70	<1	180	2	12	0	1
Rye—1 slice	70	1	150	3	16	0	13
Seven Grain—1 slice	90	1	170	4	16	0	10
Wheat—1 slice	60	1	120	3	11	0	15
White—1 slice	130	3	230	3	25	0	21